Haider Nawaf Abd Ali

The nursing role in respiratory care for COVID-19 patients

AF755317

Haider Nawaf Abd Ali

The nursing role in respiratory care for COVID-19 patients

Effect of prostrate position on dyspnea, persistent cough, and cardiopulmonary parameters among patients with covid -19

Noor Publishing

Imprint

Any brand names and product names mentioned in this book are subject to trademark, brand or patent protection and are trademarks or registered trademarks of their respective holders. The use of brand names, product names, common names, trade names, product descriptions etc. even without a particular marking in this work is in no way to be construed to mean that such names may be regarded as unrestricted in respect of trademark and brand protection legislation and could thus be used by anyone.

Cover image: www.ingimage.com

Publisher:
Noor Publishing
is a trademark of
Dodo Books Indian Ocean Ltd. and OmniScriptum S.R.L publishing group

120 High Road, East Finchley, London, N2 9ED, United Kingdom
Str. Armeneasca 28/1, office 1, Chisinau MD-2012, Republic of Moldova, Europe
Managing Directors: Ieva Konstantinova, Victoria Ursu
info@omniscriptum.com

Printed at: see last page
ISBN: 978-620-9-08133-0

Copyright © Haider Nawaf Abd Ali
Copyright © 2025 Dodo Books Indian Ocean Ltd. and OmniScriptum S.R.L publishing group

Effect of Prostrate Position and Coughing Exercises upon Level of Dyspnea, Persistent Cough, and Cardiopulmonary Parameters among Non-Intubated Patients with COVID -19

Written By

Haider Nawaf Abed Ali

List of Abbreviations and symbols

Items	*Meaning*
ACE2	Angiotensin-converting enzyme 2
Ang	Angiotensin
ALP	Alkaline phosphatase
ALT	Alanine aminotransferase
ARDS	Acute respiratory distress syndrome
AST	Aspartate aminotransferase
BP	Blood pressure
BMI	Body mass index
CK	Creatine kinase
CLIA	Chemiluminescent immunoassay
CO	Cardiac output
COPD	Chronic obstructive pulmonary disease
COVID-19	Corona Virus Disease 2019
CPAP	Continuous Positive Airway Pressure
CSI	Cough Severity index
CT scan	Computerized tomography
CVR	Content Validity Ratio
DAMPs	Damage-associated molecular pattern
DBP	Diastolic blood pressure
DI	Dyspnea index
DM	Diabetes mellitus
DVT	Deep vein thrombosis
ELISA	Enzyme-linked immunosorbent assay
f	Frequency
FiO2	Fraction of Inspired Oxygen
FVI	Face validity index
GIT	Gastrointestinal tract
GGT	Gamma-glutamyl transferase
HFNC	High flow nasal cannula
HR	Heart rate
H1N1	Swine influenza
HS	High significant
I- CVI	Item level content validity index
ICTV	International Committee on Classification of Viruses
ICU	Intensive Care Units
IEA	International Epidemiology Association
I-FVI	Item face validity index
IgA	Immunoglobulin A
IgG	Immunoglobulin G
IL	Interleukin
IgM	Immunoglobulin M
K^{th}	Distans between number and other
LDH	Lactate dehydrogenase

LMWH	Now molecular weight heparin
MAP	Mean arterial pressure
MERS	Middle east respiratory syndrom
MI	Myocardial infraction
mmHg	Milliliter mercury
ne	Number of experts in agreement
NIPPV	Non-Invasive Positive Pressure Ventilation
NS	Non-significant
$PaCO_2$	Prevalent tension of carbon dioxide
PaO_2	Partial pressure of oxygen
PE	Pulmonary embolism
PR	Pulse rate
PFT	Pulmonary function test
PP	Pulse pressure
RAAS	Renin-angiotensin-aldosterone system
RdRp	RNA-dependent RNA polymerase
RDS	Respiratory distress syndrome
RNA	Ribonucleic acid
RR	Respiratory rate
SaO2	Arterial Oxygen saturation
S	Significant
SARS-CoV-2	Severe Acute Respiratory Syndrome Coronavirus-2
SBP	Systolic blood pressure
S-CVI\Ave	Scale-level content validity index,
S-FVI	Scale face validity
SOB	Shortness of breath
SpO_2	Oxygen saturation (pulse oximetry)
UA	Universal agreement
V/Q	Ventilation perfusion
WHO	World Health Organization
↓	Decrease
↑	Increase
>	More than
<	Less than
≤	Equal or less than
%	Percent
&	And

Chapter one

Introduction

Chapter one
Introduction

1.1. Introduction:

Coronaviruses are large of family of the viruses causes many respiratory diseases range in severity from the common cold to more serious life-threatening conditions. The Coronavirus that causes the corona pandemic is a new strain that was only recently discovered on December 31st, 2019, the spread of COVID-19 began; this was confirmed by the world health organization (WHO) office in China (World Health Organization, 2020). After it is spread to other regions of China, the global alert for COVID-19 has been raised by the WHO (Ye, et al., 2020).

The COVID-19 threatens the lives of everyone in all countries of the world without exception. This impact has included the national economy of all countries, public health, trade, transport and security. This pandemic also affected the method and quality of education, as well as reduced job opportunities, thus negatively affecting individual and family income, livelihoods and entertainment. As in other crises, the most vulnerable and less economical countries with an undeveloped health system are the most influential countries in terms of the severity of infections and the number of deaths. There are also groups more exposed than others that have high risk rates due to weak immunity, mainly children, women, and the elderly (Sachs, et al., 2020).

There are four main challenges that the world's governments must face collaboratively. The first and necessary challenge is to restrain the pandemic as quickly as possible, treat cases and prevent its spread. Second challenge is the ability for meeting all an urgent and necessary need and meet them as much as possible for patients with chronic diseases, poor, elderly, and children. The third challenge is for reducing or preventing the negative change in a community health emergency into a severe financial disaster for health systems, governments, and companies. The last challenge is for rebuilding an infrastructure of health systems in a better way to be flexible, sophisticated and capable of resist health crises (Sachs, et al., 2020).

Although many of studies indicate that there was a link between most infections and wild animals, and this disease can transmitted to the human by animal, increasingly transmissions of COVID-19 from person to person by directed contact or droplet. There were also studies have indicated a rapid increase in infections and the possibility of transmissions through asymptomatic carriers, so this virus can be transmitted effectively between humans (Lai, et al., 2020).

Pneumonia associated with COVID-19 is usually severe and has peculiar phenotypes. It is characterized by severe hypoxemia and collapsed of the lung in advanced cases (Gattinoni, et al., 2020). COVID-19 pneumonia causes several problems including fever, cough, sore throat, headache, fatigue, decreasing oxygen saturation (SpO_2), and dyspnea (Zhao, et al., 2020). Also the blood pressure (BP) and pulse rate (PR) are affected with COVID-19 pneumonia (Pranata, et al., 2020).

There are two strategies to management of COVID-19 pneumonia are pharmacological and non- pharmacological. Aims of these strategies are symptomatic treatment, prevent failure of the respiratory system and other vital organs, and reduce complications and exacerbation of disease (Singhal, 2020). Non- pharmacological management of COVID-19 pneumonia increase the chance of gas exchange and improve the breathing process, in addition to reducing the effort during breathing, such as supplemental oxygen therapy, passive immunotherapy, coughing exercise, and changing the patient's position. There are several positions through which the breathing and gas exchange process can be improve, as well as reducing the effort during the inhalation and exhalation processes, and these positions are the prone and lateral position (Retucci, et al., 2020).

The application of the accurate treatment protocol and changing the position of the patient is one of the important things for the course of the treatment process; it is also the right choice for patients. There are several positions that have been prevent by studies useful to improve breathing and gas exchange, but the patient may be expose to some risks such as accidental removal of the endotracheal tube, pressure ulcers, facial edema, gastro-esophageal reflux disease, and other problems. In general, it seems that the correct choice of the patient contributes to the reduction of these complications or problems (Aeen, et al., 2021).

Imamoğlu, & Dilek, (2016), conducted study to explore the benefits of Muslim prayers and yoga on human body recommend patients for implementing the prostrate position to help them in reduce stress, flexibility, coordination and balance, in addition to strengthening immunity and strengthen their memory. In addition, the prone position is beneficial method for relief some respiratory problems. The reason for the benefit of the prone position to improve oxygenation may be due to enhancement of ventilation perfusion (V/Q) match. In this position, the dorsal side tissues are the best extended depending on the change positions with raised function of lungs residual capacity, in addition improving bronchial drainage, which increases the chance of gas exchange and makes pulmonary ventilation in good condition (Niikawa, et al., 2019).

Turning the patient's head down causes decrease in the lung stress intra-thoracic pressure, slowing the formation of lung edema, development of the disease, thus improving the breathing process, increasing the percentage of oxygen saturation, and reducing the incidence of shortness of breath (SOB) (Slessarev, et al., 2020). It is also believed that the improvement in the SpO_2 rate occurs due to the improvement of V/Q the perfusion in the prone position, because the dorsal regions (which are anatomical they have an increased number of alveolar units) it is compressed by the weight of the abdominal cavity and the mediastinum. In addition, can be reopened, resulting in employment of more efficient gas exchange areas (Coppo, et al., 2020). The prone position had effect on patients with chronic diseases; it makes to relief dyspnea and cough levels among patients with COVID-19 (Fu, et al., 2020). Also these position effects on the BP and PR (Pranata, et al., 2020).

1.2. Importance of the study:

The COVID-19 pandemic is overshadowing any health system in the world due to the huge number of patients who require intensive care for severe infection, respiratory failure, and often require intubation. Therefore, additional intervention are needed to help patients reduce mortality and help to treat or relieve moderate or severe acute respiratory distress and to achieve an effective gas exchange effect by positioning the patient appropriately for patients with pneumonia associated with COVID-19 (Coppo, et al., 2020).

Since this pandemic began to appear in China and spread to all countries of the world, it continued to increase until the number at the 22nd of February 2022 reached more than 422.000.000 confirmed cases, of which approximately 5.800.000 deaths or 1.37% attributed to the disease (World Health Organization, 2022). As for Iraq, the number of people infected with COVID-19 was up to 5th day of April 2020 is a thousand confirmed cases (Al-Mudhaffer, et al., 2020). The number continued to rise until it reached 918.155 confirmed cases and 14.678 deaths until the 10th day of April 2021. A year later, the number reached 2.303.816 confirmed cases and 24.999 deaths as of March 1st, 2022 (Ministry of Health/Environment/Public Health Department. 2022).

This pandemic is not limited to a specific age or gender, and no one is safe from it. According to the report of the WHO that 53 % of the infected are males and 47% are females, and this percentage shows that both sexes have almost the same chance of infection. The report also mentioned that the most (64%) of cases are between 25-64 years old (WHO, 2020).

The clinical effects of COVID-19 infection are highly variable. Some people with this infection remain asymptomatic, but many infected people have respiratory symptoms resulting from the pneumonia associated with this infection, and the severity of these symptoms ranges from mild to moderate, as well as severe and dangerous that leads to death. This can lead to some people needing intensive care support, especially in the elderly and those who have some chronic respiratory and immune diseases. Symptoms vary from person to person. Fever, cough, loss of smell or taste, and signs such as decrease of oxygen saturation are the first and most accessible diagnostic information. As for severe SOB, problems with gas exchange and loss of consciousness, they considered very dangerous signs, and emergency interventions must found to prevent their aggravation. The 35% of those infected with COVID-19 have a cough, while 77% of them suffer from dyspnea (Struyf, et al., 2021). Sartini, et al., (2020) reported that the most of patients had increasing in respiratory rate (RR) and decreasing in SpO_2, and Partial pressure of oxygen (PaO_2). Lee, et al., (2021) stated that the 78.75% of patients had cough, 88.26% suffering from wheezing, and 78.41% of them had dyspnea. The researcher believes, through his experience working in the COVID-19 wards, that the application prostration position and exercise of cough relieves the severity of level of dyspnea and coughing and treats some of the alterations that occur to the cardiopulmonary parameters due to corona virus 19.

1.3. The Problem statement:

The WHO announced on January 30th, 2019 a case of emergency due to the COVID-19 pandemic. In March 2020, the WHO raised the state of emergency declared COVID-19 a pandemic. In February 2020, Iraq confirmed its first cases. On April 25th, 46.135 tests were conducted in Iraq, and 1.763 positive cases were confirmed. Although Iraq is making great efforts to contain the COVID-19 pandemic by stimulating all available capabilities, complete closure and educating people about the danger of the disease. However, the number of cases and deaths began to increase significantly in June 2020. On the 2nd of July, 2020 the rate of death was about 2.2% (Alsayed, et al., 2020). According to the statement of the Ministry of Health on March 1, 2022, the number of confirmed infections in Iraq reached 2,303,816 cases, including 24.999 deaths, or 1.08% and 2.246.473 cured cases, with a rate of 95.5% (Ministry of Health / Environment / Public Health Department, 2022). Behesht, et al., (2021) reported that many clinical problems associated with COVID-19 infection causes coughing, hypoxia, dyspnea, decrease SpO_2, decrease oxygen saturation (SaO_2), decrease PaO_2, and alterations in cardiopulmonary parameters such as increase in RR, PR, and BP.

Hypoxemia is particularly perplexing to clinicians in patients with COVID-19 and is being considered. Corona virus can have a special effect on the receptors it is involved in oxygen chemo-sensitivity, so that the respiratory centers respond to low levels of oxygen, in the way the prevalent tension of carbon dioxide ($PaCO_2$). The hypoxia, effect of disease, age, and temperature-induced shifts in the whole oxygen dissociation curve contribute to the impaired brain response in controlling breathing, which makes the patient difficult to breathe (Tobin, et al., 2020). Xie, et al., (2020) recommended directing the clinical management of patients with COVID-19 requires prompt treatment of dyspnea because 25.7% of patients with SpO_2 values of 90% or less have died.

In the event that mild and moderate cases are not treated, they become cases that are more serious and may cause death, in addition to increase, the patient's stay in the hospital and these costs the health institution an additional cost and more human resources. It may make these institutions in a difficult crisis (Dawood, & Dawood, 2021). Ibraheem, et al., (2021) carried out a study to solve the problem of low SpO_2 and SOB by applying for the prone position every 3 hours. Mahrous, (2022) stated that the prone position had an effect in improving the rate of blood saturation with oxygen and reducing the heart rate and the RR to preterm neonates with respiratory distress syndrome.

The researcher believe that the other cardiopulmonary indicators had not been studied, and the position used to solve these problems may be difficult to implement every 3 hours. As the researcher think the prostrate position and coughing exercises are the optimal interventional protocol for COVID-19 patients who suffer from dyspnea, persistent cough and several cardiopulmonary parameters alterations and may be an appropriate solution to the problems discussed earlier.

1.4. Objectives of the study:

- To detect the level of dyspnea and cough among non-intubated patients with COVID-19.
- To determine the effect of prostrate position and coughing exercises upon level of dyspnea, persistent cough and cardiopulmonary parameters among non-intubated patients with COVID-19.
- To find out the relationship between the effect of prostrate position and coughing exercises upon level of dyspnea, persistent cough and cardiopulmonary parameters with participants' socio-demographic characteristics and clinical data.

1.5. Research question: Are the prostrate positions and coughing exercises able to reduce levels of dyspnea, relieve persistent cough, and improve cardiopulmonary parameters in non-intubated patients with COVID- 19?

1.6. The Study Hypothesis:

1.6.1. Null Hypothesis (H0):

1. The application of prostrate position and coughing exercise does not affect the level of dyspnea, persistent cough, and cardiopulmonary parameters among non-intubated patients with COVID -19.

1.6.2. Alternative Hypothesis (H1):

1. It is possible to relieve dyspnea and persistent cough among non-intubated patients with COVID-19 by applying the prostrate position and coughing exercises.
2. The application of the prostrate position and the practice of coughing exercises positively affect the cardiopulmonary parameters in non-intubated patients with COVID-19.

1.7. Definition of Terms:

1.7.1. Prostrate position:

A. Theoretical definition:

Defined as bending towards the ground and leaning some parts of the body on the ground so that they are equal to the position of his forehead (Salim, 2021).

B. Operational definition:

The patient with COVID-19 lies down so that his knees, forehead, and hands are close to the ground and the elbows flexed and relaxed to bear the weight of the patient. The abdominal area remains unsupported so that the position of the patient is the same as the position of prostration during prayer.

1.7.2. Coughing exercise:

A. Theoretical definition:

Is a technique used to clear the airway of secretion or sputum by facilitating the excretion of excessive secretion from the distal part of the lung (Urme, et al., 2019).

B. Operational Definition: Is a technique done by patients with COVID-19 that is carried out by taking a deep breath, calmly and without effort, and

then holding the breath for two or three seconds and exhaling it forcefully in the form of a repeated cough to remove all secretions.

1.7.3. Dyspnea:

A. Theoretical Definition:

Known as an uncomfortable or unpleasant feeling or sensation during breathing so that this symptom has many negatives, including physical, emotional and psychosocial effects (Kako, et al., 2018).

B. Operational Definition:

A case of difficulty of breathing that makes the patients with COVID-19 resort to using the abdominal muscles and making an extra effort during the breathing process. Therefore, the process of inhalation and exhalation becomes a strenuous and exhausting process for these patients.

1.7.4. Cough:

A. Theoretical Definition: A defensive reflex that helps to clear of secretions and sputum from the airways and prevent aspiration of foreign materials to the lower airways (De Blasio, et al., 2011).

B. Operational Definition: A condition that occurs in patients with COVID-19 characterized by scratching the airway due to the presence of secretions and often accompanied by SOB, which causes the patient to exhale air in the form of a frequent cough.

1.7.5. Cardiopulmonary parameters:

A. Theoretical Definition:

Measurement of certain things that indicates to functions and work that related to the heart and lungs (Dox, et al 2001).

B. Operational Definition:

Are a list of indicators refers to the function of the heart and lungs that will be measured and followed up for patients with COVID-19 and these indicators include: systolic blood pressure (SBP), diastolic blood pressure (DBP), pulse pressure (PP), PR, cardiac output (CO), mean arterial pressure (MAP), RR, and SpO_2.

Chapter two

Review of Literature

Chapter Two
Review of Literature

Outline of Review of Literature:

2.1. Overview of the COVID-19:

2.2. Historical aspect of the COVID-19:

2.3. Risk factors associated with COVID-19:

2.4. Pathophysiology of COVID-19:

2.5. Clinical manifestations of COVID-19:

2.6. Diagnostic tests of COVID-19:

2.7. Complications associated with COVID-19:

2.8. Therapeutic management of patient with COVID-19:

- 2.8.1. Non-pharmacological management:
  - 2.8.1. a. Supplement oxygen therapy:
  - 2.8.1. b. Positioning:
  - 2.8.1. c. Passive immunotherapy:
  - 2.8.1. d. Cough management:
  - 2.8.1. e. Intubation and mechanical ventilation:
- 2.8.2. Pharmacological management:
  - 2.8.2. a. Anti-viral drugs:
  - 2.8.2. b. Antibiotics drugs:
  - 2.8.2. c. Dexamethasone:
  - 2.8.2. d. Antipyretic drug:
  - 2.8.2. e. Anticoagulant drugs:
  - 2.8.2.f. Immune boosting against COVID-19:

2.9. Benefits of positioning for patient with COVID-19:

- 2.9.1. The effect of position on severity of dyspnea and persistent cough:
- 2.9.2. The effect of position on cardiopulmonary parameters:

2.10. Benefits of coughing exercises on severity of dyspnea, persistent cough, and cardiopulmonary parameters:

2.11. Theoretical framework:

2.12. Previous related studies:

2.1. Overview about COVID-19:

The WHO defines COVID-19 as a newly emerging pandemic disease that spreads globally. A pandemic is the emerging or developing of a new disease and its transformation to spread throughout the world and on a very large area and affect a large number of people, this is the most accepted definition of the word pandemic by the International Epidemiology Association (IEA). Pandemic have two types of risks, the first 'Spark risk' linked to the origin of the outbreak, the second is "risk spread" and this is how likely it is to spread through humans and here lies the seriousness of the pandemic (Seneviwickrama, et al., 2020).

COVID-19 is a severe acute respiratory syndrome that appeared in the city of Wuhan in China's Hubei Province in late 2019 spread outside China to infect all countries of the world. Being a new strain of coronavirus, it was later named novel coronavirus 2019 (n COV- 2019) (Wu, 2020). COVID-19: is a newly discovered strain of coronavirus that causes acute respiratory syndrome. So that the WHO recognized on January 12, 2020, after confirming the spread of the virus outside China, that the origin of the disease is the Corona virus and is called COVID-19 (Bassareo, et al., 2020).

2.2. History of COVID-19:

In December 2019, a new pandemic disease characterized by rapid growth and onset, later called Coronavirus disease 2019 (COVID-19), causes terror and fear in the people all over the world due to the high number of deaths and the number of cases (Morens, et al., 2020). Similar to the 20th century, the 21th century has seen many pandemics of the flu strain, which are:

- Severe acute respiratory syndrome corona virus (SARS-COV): first appeared in 2003 in China in Guangdong region (Demiray, 2021).

- Swine flu or influenza A (H1N1): is the first pandemic of the twenty-first century, which appeared in 2009 in Mexico and the United States of America (USA) and spread to large areas of the world (Seneviwickrama, et al., 2020).
- Middle Eastern Respiratory Syndrome Coronavirus (MERS-COV): is the first emerged in 2012 in Saudi Arabia (Demiray, 2021).
- Corona Virus Disease 2019 (COVID-19): A newly series of severe respiratory infection cases appeared in December 2019, in Wuhan, Hubei County, China. (Bassareo, et al., 2020).
- Omicron: The WHO announced the discovery of the omicron strain in Johannesburg, South Africa on November 26, 2021(Petersen, et al., 2022).

2.3 Risk factors of COVID-19:

There are several risk factors, whether demographic or social factors, or previous diseases, all of which contribute to increasing the severity and risk of infection with COVID- 19. These include smoking, obesity, elderly person (> 65 years old), diabetes mellitus (DM), and pre-existing cardiovascular diseases: hypertension, atherosclerosis, stroke, myocardial infraction (MI), pre-existing respiratory diseases such as chronic obstructive pulmonary disease (COPD) and asthma (Singh, et al., 2021).

2.4. Pathophysiology of COVID-19:

2.4.1. Viral Invasion:

Chemically, the corona virus that causes COVID-19 consists of four main structural glycoproteins: they are spike (S), membrane (M), envelope (E), and nucleocapsid (N) as figure (2-1). The specific function of the three proteins M, E and N is to assemble and release viral particles, while the function of the S protein is responsible for viral binding and entry into host cells. This S protein needs a receptor to help it enter the cell. The angiotensin-converting enzyme 2 (ACE2) acts as an entry receptor for SARS-COV2 (Bohn, 2020 and Felsenstein, et al., 2020).

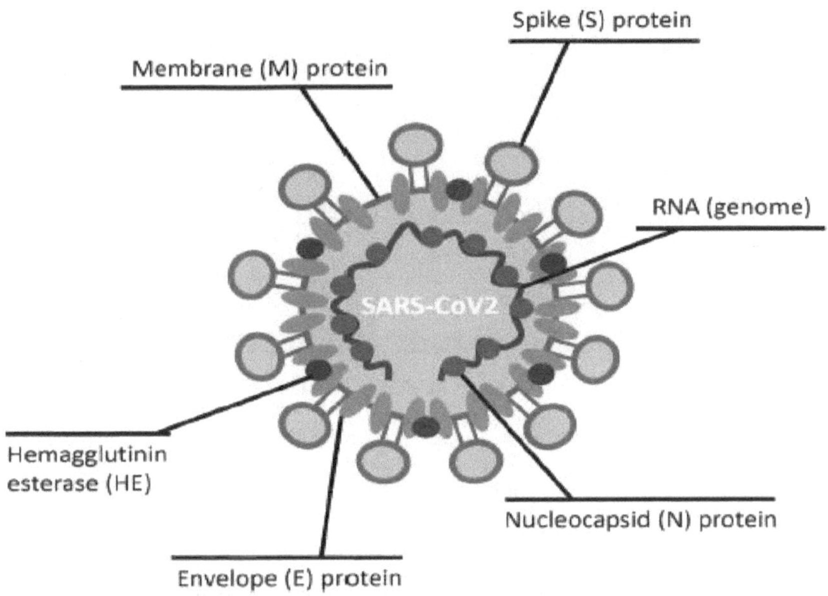

Figure (2-1): Chemical structure of SARS cov2 virus (Felsenstein, et al., 2020).

Sever acute respiratory syndrome coronavirus 2 (SARSCOV2) is transmitted through large respiratory droplets that directly enter cells of the upper part of the respiratory system, especially the nasal ciliary and lower respiratory tract as the alveolar epithelial cells of the lungs (figure 2-2). the ACE2 is also expressed in many other human tissues, such as heart, kidneys, thyroid gland, and small intestine fatty tissues as well as the testicle, and this gives an opportunity to infect this virus to organs other than the lungs directly when a case of viremia occurs. Viral and cellular membranes fuse with each other after the host cell attaches, facilitating virus entry into the cell (Bohn, 2020).

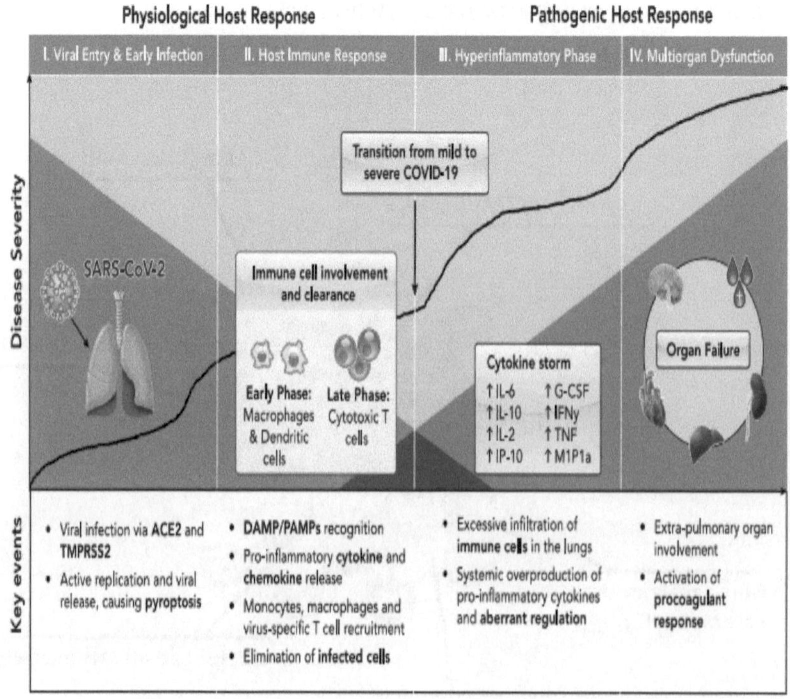

Figure (2-2): Pathophysiological progression status in COVID-19 (Bohn, 2020).

2.4.2 Initial physiological immune response:

If the immune system is in good condition and well-coordinated, it will present the desired response as the first line of physiology defense against SARS-COV2 infection. Infection with COVID- 19 leads to cell death and injury to airway epithelial cells (Bohn, 2020).

2.4.3. Prominent changes in hematology and coagulation:

When the SARS-COV2 enters the body, it binds to ACE2; it is the natural receptor and helps it enter the cell. After the virus enters the cell, it damages the alveolar epithelium in the alveoli and causes damage to its lining, which shows us the common respiratory symptoms associated with COVID-19 (Levi, & Thachil, 2020). There is another opinion about the occurrence of thrombosis associated with COVID-19, which is that the virus triggers a so-called "cytokine storm", which contributes to damage to the blood vessels through the occurrence of local inflammation, which obliges leukocytes and macrophage cells / monocytes to be present in the affected area, which can be it then exacerbates local inflammation, cell injury, and endothelial damage and activation of coagulation, which in turn leads to the consumption of clotting factors and accelerated fibrinolysis. Finally, it can be said that blood clots occur after the exacerbation of the inflammatory processes associated with infection with COVID-19. These clots can occur in small vessels in several organs other than the lungs, such as the heart, kidneys, liver, and pancreas (Christensen, et al., 2020).

2.5. Clinical manifestations of COVID-19:

COVID-19 lead to many different clinical manifestations that vary in severity from one person to another, so it is asymptomatic in some infected cases, moderate in many of them, and severe and fatal in a few cases. The most common clinical manifestations of COVID-19 are dyspnea, fever, cough, muscle weakness, sore throat, and chest pain. There are also less frequent symptoms such as taste and olfactory problems, cardiac, gastrointestinal, neurological, dermatological, and rheumatic manifestations as shown in figure (2-3) (Baj, et al., 2020). In this study, we will review all the clinical manifestations associated with COVID-19 according to the different body systems as follow:

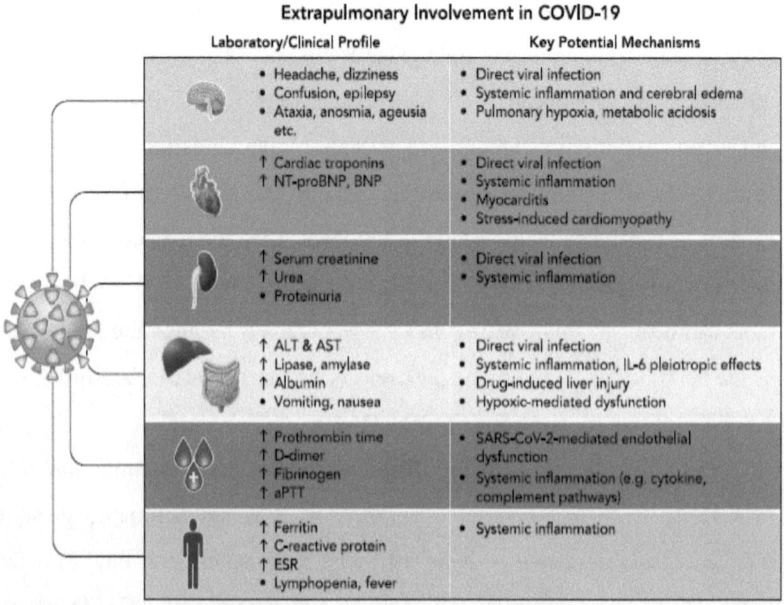

Figure (2-3): Extra pulmonary clinical manifestations and key potential mechanisms noted in the severe COVID-19 patients (Bohn, et al., 2020)

2.5.1. Respiratory clinical features in COVID-19:

Many clinical signs and symptoms have appeared, although they differ from one person to another, but they occur in most patients infected with the emerging corona virus. The respiratory system has the largest proportion of complications and the occurrence of problems, including the most serious clinical manifestations from COVID- 19 such as fever and cough, dyspnea and hypoxia, which lead to severe respiratory failure (George, 2020).

2.5.1. a. Dyspnea and hypoxemia associated with COVID-19:

So far, the relationship between dyspnea and COVID- 19 is unknown. However, all studies indicate that dyspnea is present in COVID- 19 patients as one of the infection problems, and may come with some neurological symptoms due to the presence of common underlying pathogenic mechanisms. Dyspnea is present in the 31.8% of patients with COVID- 19 (Ora, et al., 2020). In COVID-19, hypoxemia may occur with or without dyspnea. A change in lung compliance does not mean an inevitable sign of hypoxemia. However, severe hypoxemia remains a life-threatening sign (Swenson, et. al., 2021). Despite the confirmation of the presence of hypoxemia and pneumonia associated with COVID-19 infection, but the possibility remains that the occurrence of dyspnea is related to the effect of neuropathy caused by infection with the COVID-19 virus (Matschke, 2020). There are several causes of hypoxemia in COVID-19 that are as follow:

2.5.1.a.1. Intrapulmonary shunting:

Infection with COVID-19 leads to mild localized pulmonary edema which results in ground glass opacity and coherence on chest imaging, surfactant loss and superimposed pressure, resulting in alveolar collapse and a significant decrease in CO of non-aerated perfusion of lung tissue, leading to intrapulmonary shunt (Gattinoni, et al., 2020).

2.5.1.a.2. Loss of lung perfusion regulation: After COVID-19 infection, pathophysiological changes in that include:

- Relative failure of the hypoxic pulmonary vasoconstriction mechanism (constriction of the small pulmonary arteries in response to alveolar hypoxia) (Archer, et al., 2020). To treat this failure, the body needs to secrete prostaglandins (an endogenous dilator), bradykinin, and cytokines associated with the inflammatory process (Dhont, et al., 2020).
- A defect in the regulation of renin-angiotensin aldosterone system (RAAS) , ACE2 itself acts as a major functional receptor for SARS-COV2 to enter the cell and this is what we mentioned earlier, since ACE2 converts angiotensin II to angiotensin 1-7 which is also important for reducing bradykinin. Thus, pulmonary vasoconstriction occurs due to an increase in angiotensin II resulting from decreased levels of ACE2 enzyme (Zhang, & Baker, 2017).

2.5.1.a.3. Intravascular micro thrombi:

COVID-19 infection directly affects pulmonary capillary endothelial cells that express ACE2. The occurrence of micro thrombi inside the blood vessels is the end result is due to an imbalance between pro-coagulant and fibrinolytic activity in the presence of acute inflammation, or it could be due to inhibition of plasminogen activation and fibrinolysis by increased activity of plasminogen activator inhibitor which are stimulated as proteins in the acute phase of the disease. Patients with COVID-19 develop elevated dimers, which indicate the formation of blood clots. Therefore, D-dimer levels are checked to predict the occurrence of thrombosis in the blood vessels. The occurrence of micro thrombi within the pulmonary vasculature also causes ventilation perfusion (V/Q) mismatch and lung tissue damage (Bikdeli, 2020).

2.5.1. b. Cough associated with COVID-19:

Cough is one of the annoying symptoms of COVID-19, as it causes other harmful symptoms such as chest pain, fatigue, SOB and cognitive impairment. This is a group of long-term effects referred to as post-covid syndrome, or long-term covid syndrome. After infected with SARS-COV2, the invasion of vagal sensory neurons and a neuro-inflammatory response are occurring. That led peripheral and central hypersensitivity of cough pathways which causes COVID-19 cough occur as shown in figure (2-4) (Song, et al., 2021). Coughing occurs in 33% of young people infected with the Coronavirus, while it occurs in the elderly by 40%. This indicates that coughing occurs in all age groups in similar proportions (Liu, et al., 2020). While a study was conducted in China by Zhu, et al., (2020), reported that 3062 patients infected with COVID-19, about 63% of patients with COVID- 19 were suffered from cough. In Iraq, Al-Mudhaffer, et al., (2020) conducted a study to show the clinical symptoms of COVID-19 for 1153 patients, reported that 44.4% of patient with COVID-19 were suffering from cough.

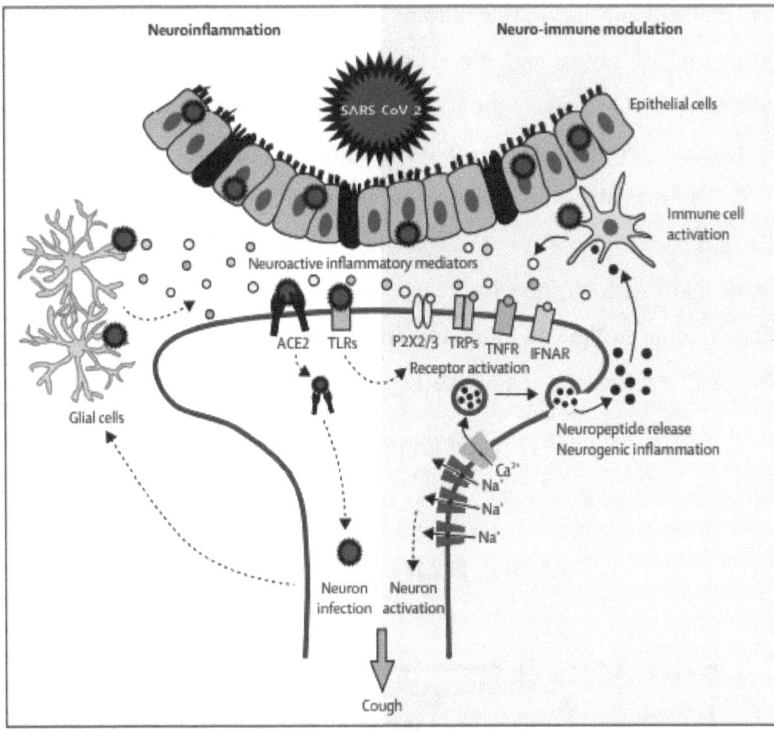

Figure (2- 4): cough mechanisms in SARS-COV2 infection (Song, et al., 2021).

2.5.2 Cardiovascular clinical features in COVID-19:

Because of the rapid spread of the COVID-19 virus among people, that makes prevention and alleviation of its complications very difficult. Although the clinical respiratory signs and symptoms associated with COVID-19 are prominent and clear, there are other clinical symptoms that accompany COVID-19, including those related to cardiovascular symptoms, which we will address some of it as follow:

2.5.2.1. Hypertension: As we mentioned earlier, at the beginning of the infection with Covid19, the SARS COV2 uses ACE2 as its receptor to help it enter the cell via spike protein. This association causes a disturbance in the RAAS. After this link, a deficiency of ACE2 occurs, whether inside or outside the lung. Since ACE2 contributes to the conversion of angiotensin 2 to angiotensin 1-7, the latter binds to the MAS-R receptor, which acts as an anti-inflammatory, Anti-fibrotic, Nitric Oxide, and Vasodilation. The loss of ACE2 causes high blood pressure, respiratory distress, and fibrosis after SARS COV2 enters the cell as it contributes to the increased spread of inflammation (South, et al., 2020). High blood pressure may be associated with 2.5 times higher risk of severe and fatal COVID- 19, especially among the elderly (Lippi, et al., 2020). High blood pressure has a significant association with an increase in the severity of COVID- 19 infection and deterioration in the condition and an increase in mortality rates as shown Figure (2-5) (Pranata, et al., 2020).

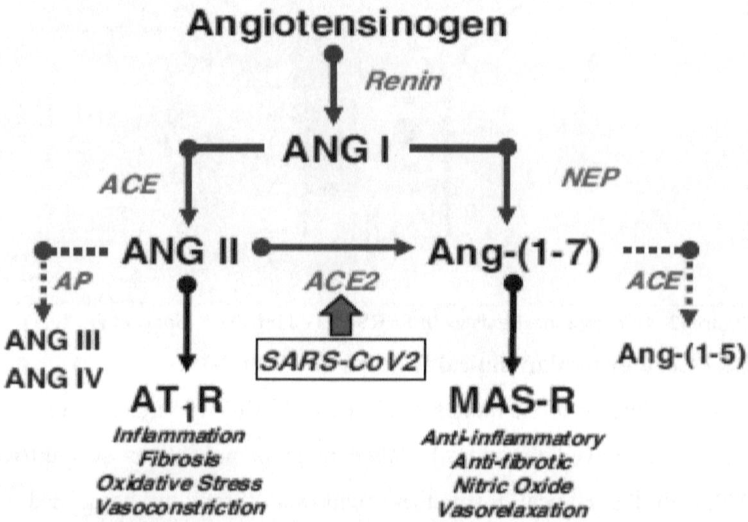

Figure (2-5): Renin- Angiotensin- Aldosterone System (RAAS) (South, et al., 2020).

2.5.2.2. Hypotension:

After entering SARS cov2 inside the cell, by using ACE2 as its receptor, which helps it enter the pulmonary cell, the need for ACE2 may be reduced therefore, an increase in angiotensin 1-7 to which the MAS-R receptor that is vasodilation binds, causes blood pressure disorder resulting in a relative hypotension that can occur in patients with COVID-19 in later stages of the disease (South, et al., 2020).

2.5.2.3. Tachycardia: Some studies have indicated that SARS COV2 increases the activity of the cytokine that causes an increase in metabolic rate and this requires increased work on the heart, similar to influenza (Kwong, et al., 2018).

2.5.2.4. Thrombus formation:

Severe inflammation caused by SARS COV2, which may lead to destabilization of vascular plaques, and because it increases coagulation activity, thus increasing the risk of thrombosis of blood vessels, whether inside or outside the lung (Mehta, et al., 2020).

2.5.3 Gastrointestinal clinical features in COVID-19:

Although COVID-19 is a respiratory disease and is transmitted and reproduced through the respiratory system, the digestive system is the secondary site for the spread of SARS-COV2 virus because it also contains ACE2, which is the natural receptor of the virus. SARS-COV2 causes many gastrointestinal (GIT) symptoms, including nausea, vomiting, anorexia, diarrhea, abdominal pain, elevated blood glucose levels, and elevated liver function tests that include aspartate aminotransferase (AST), alanine transaminase (ALT), gamma-glutamyl tansferase (GGT), and alkaline phosphatase (ALP) as shown figure (2-6) (Pola, et al., 2021). The symptoms of the digestive system associated with COVID-19 occur in varying proportions, include abdominal pain occurs in 3% of people with COVID-19, while nausea, vomiting, and diarrhea occur in rates of 21%, 14%, and 46%, respectively (Zhou, et al., 2020) 83.8% suffer from anorexia and 22.2% have impaired liver function (Pan, et al., 2020).

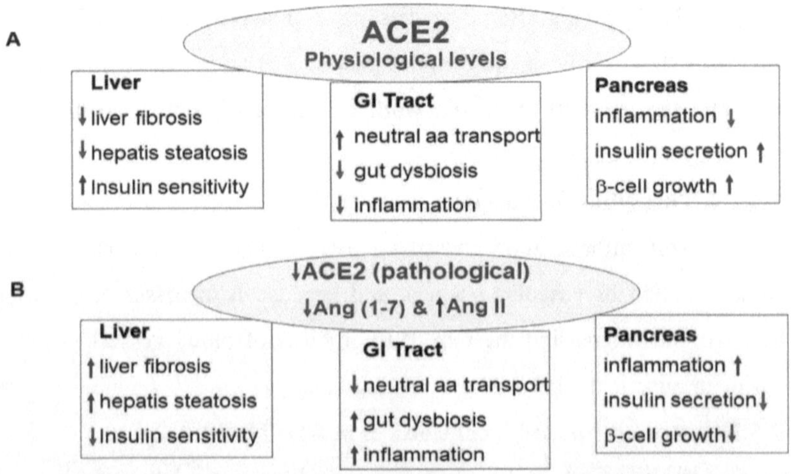

Figure (2-6): The role of ACE2 in GIT physiology and pathology caused by COVID-19 (Pola, et al., 2021).

2.5.4 Dermatological clinical features in COVID-19:

The receptor for SARS -COV2 is ACE2, which has been shown to be secreted from many tissues in the human body, including adipose tissue and skin. Therefore, some patients show skin symptoms accompanying the infection with COVID-19, which are itching, chilblain-like eruption, pruritus, erythematous-edematous lesions, urticarial rash, petechia, chickenpox-like rashes, maculopapular rash, mottling, pityriasis rosea-like eruptions, palmar erythema, bullous eruption (Wollina, et al., 2020), ecchymosis of the fingers and toes, acro-ischemia, atopic dermatitis, eruptive cherry angioma, undefined margins, bleaching, mostly located at the neck, trunk, back, and proximal portions of upper and lower limbs (Criado, et al., 2020), papulovesicular, dry gangrene, ulcer (Li, et al., 2020). A study conducted by Recalcati, (2020) showed that skin symptoms of COVID-19 occur at a rate of 20.4%, of which 15.9% are erythematous rash and 1.1% for chickenpox-like vesicles and 3.4% for urticaria. Galván, et al., (2020) conducted a study involving 429 patients with COVID- 19, 92% of whom had pruritus, 15% of vesicular lesions, and 56% of maculopapular lesions. Duong, et al., (2020) reported that 28.5% of

COVID- 19 patients who developed skin symptoms had exanthema, 14.2% had chicken pox like vesicles, and 7% had urticaria.

2.5.5 Neurological clinical features in COVID-19:

Many neurological symptoms that may appear on some patients with COVID -19, which are headache, malaise, unstable walking, languidness, cerebral hemorrhage, cerebral infarction, dizziness impaired consciousness (Wang, et al., 2020). Hyposmia is not a total loss of smell, but a reduced ability to smell and to detect odors, hypogeusia is a reduced ability to taste things (to taste sweet, sour, bitter, or salty substances) (Nouchi, et al., 2021). Stroke, and seizures (Lahiri, & Ardila, 2020), myalgia (muscle pain) (Orsucci, et al., 2020), are another neurological signs and symptoms that result from COVID-19 infection.

2.5.6 Urinary and reproductive system clinical features in COVID-19:

The SARS COV2 virus is capable of infecting the urinary system and causing functional and physiological damages in it like the rest of the other body systems, and is not limited to the respiratory system only. Studies have indicated that ACE2 is not only present in alveolar cells, but it has also been shown to be present in urinary system, including cells of the proximal renal tubules, urinary bladder cells , as well as males reproductive system, including leydig and cells in the seminal ducts in the testis. Because this virus invades the cells of the urinary system, it results in a number of symptoms and problems that are specific to this system, including urinary tract infection, mild proteinuria, hematuria, elevated serum creatinine, and elevated urea nitrogen (Wu, et al., 2020).

2.5.7. Fever:

Fever is an increase in core body temperature that exceeds normal limit hypothalamus thermoregulation. The most common cause of fever is brain dysfunction caused by infection and sepsis. The effect of fever on patients infected with COVID-19 is varying severity and incidence. The mechanism of the occurrence of high body temperature associated with COVID-19 is not without one of the following three reasons:

- Direct brain infected with SARS COV2, it causes a defect in hypothalamus thermoregulation.
- Persistent immune defect or disorder resulting from SARS COV2 invasion, which results in a defect in the regulation of cytokines and an increase in their secretion.
- Thrombosis of blood vessels (Suwanwongse, & Shabarek, 2020).

2.6. Diagnostic test of COVID-19:

Since the WHO announced the spread of a new pandemic in the world, which is COVID-19 in 2020, and so far, the world has not agreed on determining the appropriate diagnostic tests for COVID-19, which led to the occurrence of confusion among healthcare professionals about determine test priorities and interpret results. However, scientists did not stand idly by about this pandemic, but studies indicated some previously known diagnostic tests that can identify and diagnose COVID-19 infection at a high rate. Opinions differ in studies on COVID-19 about the incubation period from infection to first symptoms. Almost all researchers agreed that the incubation period for COVID-19 is typically 5-7 days, with a range of 4-14 days (Beeching, et al., 2020). There are many common tests that are used today to diagnose COVID-19, including:

2.6.1. The reverse transcriptase polymerase chain reaction (RT- PCR):

Because of advances in nuclear medical diagnosis virus detection and diagnosis is made easy using quick and easy acid detection techniques. Considered PCR the "gold standard" for detecting some viruses because it is characterized by rapid detection and high sensitivity and quality. This technology has become it helps us a lot in diagnosing early infection of SARS COV2.This procedure is carried out by making a nasal swab and throat swab and examining them to detect the presence of acids specific to SARS cov2 (Tahamtan & Ardebili, 2020).

2.6.2. The Chemiluminescent immunoassay (CLIA):

Is a modified version of Enzyme-linked immunosorbent assay (ELISA) where luminescence is measured for the detection of pathogens. It is a quantitative test that can measure the number of immunoglobulin G (IgG), immunoglobulin M (IgM), and immunoglobulin A (IgA) antibodies. This test allows the mixing of patient samples with viral specific proteins. The formation of the antigen-antibody complex is then detected by the binding of another secondary antibody that undergoes a chemical reaction for producing light. The amount of emitted light is then calculated for measuring the number of antibodies present in the sample. Only two days after the onset of fever is enough for the detection of IgG. But IgM cannot be detected before the detection of IgG (Cai, et al., 2020).

2.6.3. Rapid diagnostic tests (RDT):

This examination needs a time ranging between 10-30 minutes. The mechanism of it is to work on principle of the lateral flow assay where the antibody to antigen is the compound moves through the action of capillaries across the membrane and is immobilized by capturing antibodies by the appearance of colored lines confirm the presence of a detectable titer of IgM and IgG antibodies that binds to virus particles, in other words, it works to determine the presence or absence of antibodies against the virus in the patient's blood serum samples, as it cannot count the number of antibodies in the blood sample (Asrani, 2021).

2.6.4. Ultrasonography: After studies have proven an increased incidence of deep vein thrombosis (DVT) and blood clotting in vital organs such as the heart, lungs and brain as a result of infection with COVID-19, there have been calls for the use of full-body ultrasound for patients with COVID-19 (Zhang, 2020).

2.6.5. Lung computed tomography (CT) scan:

Since the emergence of the COVID-19 pandemic until now, there has been a divergence of opinions about diagnostic methods. But the CT scan of the lung remains the agreed upon examination to determine the severity of pneumonia associated with Covid-19 by detecting ground glass opacity in reticular pattern and crazy paving pattern (Shah, et al., 2021).

2.6.6. Chest-X-ray:

Chest x-ray technology remains one of the easy to use techniques available in all health institutions, but it does not give specific and accurate results in detecting infection with the COVID-19 virus, x- ray can differentiate between normal results, pneumonia and COVID-19. Patchy ground glass opacity in an infected person's lung is evidence of COVID-19 diagnoses (Mangal, et al., 2020).

2.7. Complications associated with COVID-19:

Because it is a new pandemic, there is not enough and conclusive information so far about the possible complications of this disease. However, some studies have discovered physiological changes associated with COVID-19 in some of the patient's cells that may cause rapid complications due to the exacerbation of COVID-19 infection. These changes include endothelial dysfunction in the pulmonary blood vessels, and this may later lead to pulmonary thrombosis or pulmonary embolism (PE) (George, et al., 2020).

2.7.1. Respiratory complications of COVID-19:

- When SARS-COV2 enters the alveoli, specifically the alveolar epithelium, which it secretes ACE2 , that is the natural receptor for the virus to help it to enter the lung cell and thus SARS COV2 destroys and damages tissues as shown figure (2-7) (Brosnahan, et al., 2020).

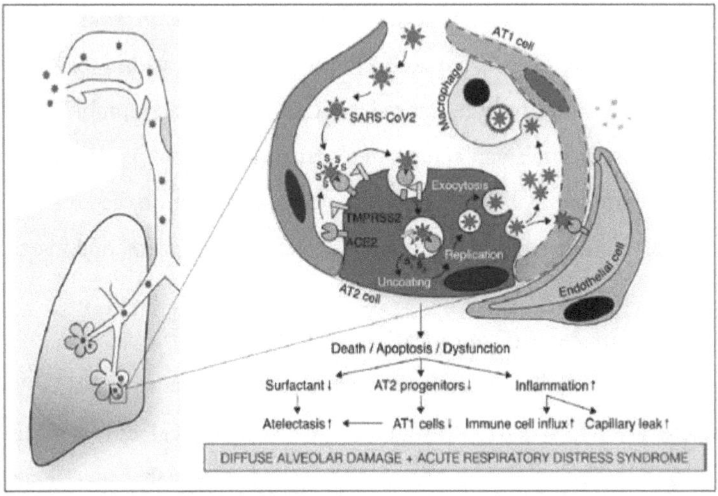

Figure (2-7): The pathological implications of SARS-COV2 infection on alveolar epithelial injury (Brosnahan, et al., 2020).

- Pulmonary micro-vascular thrombosis: Some studies have indicated that approximately 27% of patients admitted to intensive care units who suffer from pneumonia associated with COVID-19 have venous thromboembolic disease. All of them had high levels of fibrinogen, D-dimer, and platelet counts. And these patients had high rates of death (Brosnahan, et al., 2020).
- Diaphragm disuse atrophy: Mechanical ventilation is important to assist the breathing of unconscious patients and those with respiratory failure or other respiratory conditions. But at the same time, there are negative effects of mechanical ventilation on the respiratory system, including inactivity and atrophy of the diaphragm due to its inactivity (Dres, et al., 2017).

2.7.2. Cardiovascular complications of COVID-19: After entering the various cells of the body SARS-COV2 causes disruption in the regulation of the immune system, increased metabolism and inflammatory processes of the lining of blood vessels which may lead to destabilization of vascular plaques, causing blood clots, as well as this virus increases the activity of cytokines that cause increased metabolism, which leads to increased demand on the heart, similar to influenza. The virus may also cause direct damage to the heart using ACE2 receptors located within the heart tissue. Because of the damage caused by this virus, many problems with the cardiovascular system appear, including myocardial injury, myocarditis, acute coronary syndrome, acute myocardial infarction, acute heart failure and cardiomyopathy, dysrhythmias, venous thromboembolic event (Long, et al., 2020).

2.7.3. Neurological complications of COVID-19:

Despite the widespread morbidity and mortality of COVID-19 but there are a few studies examining the neurological effects of infection caused by SARS-COV-2. But there are some studies that have reviewed the neurological complications of this disease, including meningitis, septic encephalopathy, delirium, ischemic stroke due to hypercoagulability, and hypoxic encephalopathy (Sheraton, et al., 2020).

2.7.4. Urinary and reproductive system complications of COVID-19:

Since renal cells share with lung, heart and other cells in the expression of ACE2 and since there is a close link between SARS COV2 and ACE2, there must be kidney damage as a result of this virus entering those cells. These damages or complications include: severe acute kidney injury, renal failure (rare), viral orchitis, decreased testosterone hormone secretion, and subclinical hypogonadism (Jin, et al., 2021).

2.8. Therapeutic management of COVID-19:

The treatment guidelines for COVID-19 vary between countries, to date; there is no standardized and approved treatment. However, some experimental clinical studies indicated that there is a response of this disease to some therapeutic techniques that reduce the severity of the disease and reduce mortality (Tobaiqy, et al., 2020).

2.8.1. Non-pharmacological management:

Non-pharmacological interventions to treat some signs and symptoms are among the most important duties of the nurse.

2.8.1. a. Supplement oxygen therapy:

One of the most important challenges facing COVID-19 patients and health care workers is the functional deterioration of the respiratory system and its failure resulting from the pneumonia associated with COVID-19. These challenges are especially high in underdeveloped countries that do not have a sufficient number of beds in intensive care units (Smit, et al., 2020).

Oxygen can be lifesaving and reduce disease progression, severity and complications oxygen therapy is used to treat early hypoxia in patients with SOB. Supplemental oxygen therapy is used in different ways. If the patient is conscious, oxygen can be used with non-surgical options, including a face mask, high flow nasal cannula (HFNC), continuous positive airway pressure (CPAP) and non-invasive positive pressure ventilation (NIPPV) should be considered. But if the patient is unconscious, intubation is the best solution to provide the patient with oxygen (Gattinoni, et al., 2020).

2.8.1. b. Positioning:

Patients suffering from SOB should take position conserve energy while allowing maximum lung expansion. These patients cannot tolerate lying down and in the spinal position. They must take the comfortable position for the respiratory system, such as the Fowler or semi-fowler position that keeps the contents of the abdomen from congestion in the lungs or sitting on a chair while bending forward and putting it down elbows on their knees or a table over the bed (tripod position) or other positions (Williams & Hopper, 2015). The prone position has been suggested as an unconventional treatment for hypoxemia in life-threatening situations. The prone position improves the pulmonary gas exchange and breathing process by repositioning the heart to the chest to recruit the pulmonary alveoli, and improving ventilation perfusion (Pereira, et al., 2021).

2.8.1. c. Passive immunotherapy:

Passive immunotherapy is made from human plasma, usually containing more than 95% unmodified IgG. Passive immunotherapy based on monoclonal antibodies is an effective method for treating and relieving symptoms of infectious diseases. Hence, it becomes an alternative in the treatment of COVID-19. Antibodies in human plasma directed at the MERS spike protein, it showed promising results in vitro and in vivo, which demonstrated clinical improvement for COVID-19 patients after passive immunotherapy (Pereira, et al., 2021).

2.8.1. d. Cough management:

Coughing can be treated without medication by following the nurse's instructions by applying the following steps-:

- Close your mouth or place your hand over your mouth and swallow once immediately after feeling a cough or tickle that occurs in the pharynx area.
- Keep your hand over your mouth or keep it closed and hold your breath for a few seconds and breathe in through your nose very slowly.
- If the cough stops or decreases in frequency, breathe deeply and slowly through the nose only and keep your hand away from the mouth.
- In the case of persistent coughing or persistent tickling in the throat you must repeat the application of the previous steps until the cough stops or relieves (Berman, et al., 2016).

2.8.1. e. Intubation and mechanical ventilation:

Endotracheal intubation is an urgent intervention that involves inserting a flexible tube of appropriate size in the trachea to keep the airway open and provide ventilation. Some cases, such as unconsciousness, major operations, severe hypoxia, partial or total airway blockage such as laryngospasm, or respiratory disorders including ARDS and COVID-19, may need this technique. Intubation is uncomfortable technique that is usually done under general anesthesia with the use of neuromuscular-blocking medications. Some patients develop severe respiratory distress and respiratory failure during the COVID-19 pandemic; these patients require intubation immediately to avoid diseases progression (Mohammadi, et al., 2021).

2.8.2. Pharmacological management:

No official registered treatment for COVID-19 has been announced. However, there are treatments that rely mainly on supportive therapy and on symptomatic treatment, in an attempt to prevent failure of the respiratory system and other vital organs, as well as to reduce complications and exacerbation of disease (Singhal, 2020).

2.8.2. a. Anti-viral medications:

2.8.2. a.1. Remdesivir:

Previous clinical trial studies were conducted on this treatment and it was found that it is effective on the viral polymerase enzyme of coronaviruses, so SARS and MERS patients were treated with it. Now, some studies of COVID-19 patients in China have used it, and the results of its work are that it works by incorporation into the nascent viral RNA chain and then causing its early termination (Al-Tawfiq, et al., 2020).

2.8.2. a.2. Chloroquine / Hydroxychloroquine:

Hydroxychloroquine is a drugs used to treat malaria and amebiasis. Some studies have shown that it has a positive effect in the treatment of SARS and avian flu. It is considered an antiviral through an increase in the internal pH necessary for the fusion between the virus and the host cell. It is also affects ACE2 receptors. Recent studies have shown evidence of its effectiveness in COVID-19 patients. As studies indicated, hydroxychloroquine in vitro is stronger than Chloroquine in SARS-COV-2 inhibition (Wang, al., 2020).

2.8.2.a.3. Favipiravir:

Is a selective and potent inhibitor of RNA-dependent RNA polymerase (RdRp) of RNA viruses. Favipiravir is incorporated into the nascent viral RNA by error prone viral RdRp, which leads to chain termination and viral mutagenesis. Favipiravir is a broad-spectrum oral medication. Reports of in vitro studies have shown that Favipiravir can have an effective effect against SARS-COV-2 infection. Favipiravir has been approved in many countries as a drug already approved for COVID-19 pandemic (Joshi, 2020).

2.8.2. b. Antibiotics medications:

2.8.2.b.1. Azithromycin: Has shown to regulate cytokines, maintain epithelial cell integrity or prevent lung fibrosis. Azithromycin was used to viral infections other than COVID-19 have been reported and its use has been associated with lower mortality and ventilation days. Specialists used this drug for patients with COVID-19 to treat secondary infections of the respiratory tract associated with COVID-19. It has been shown to be beneficial throughout its use during the treatment period. However, the evidence for its use is not yet sufficient (Echeverría-Esnal, et al., 2021).

2.8.2.b.2. Other Antibiotics medications:

Infection with COVID-19 exposes the patient to secondary problems represented by multiple functional and physiological damages, including pneumonia accompanying COVID-19, which may lead to respiratory failure and injury to the heart muscle, whether due to infections or other damages such as cardiac arrhythmias as well as injury to other body organs such as the liver, kidneys, pancreas, brain, and others. In addition, infections that accompany COVID-19 infection occur in different parts of the body, it is necessary to use antibiotics to treat these infections, reduce damage and prevent the failure of multiple organs through the use of one of the following antibiotics: Meropenem, moxifloxacin, levofloxacin, Vancomycin, and ceftriaxone sodium (Du, et al., 2020).

2.8.2. c. Dexamethasone:

Dexamethasone is a glucocorticoid that was previously used to treat respiratory problems during various respiratory infections. Some studies have shown that dexamethasone reduces mortality by 30% for COVID-19 patients who undergo mechanical ventilation and 20% for those who need oxygen without mechanical ventilation. Studies have also shown that dexamethasone has not given good results in patients who do not need ventilation. However, one of the disadvantages of dexamethasone is that it suppresses the immune system and can thus potentially exacerbate viral infections (Chakraborty, & Parvez, 2020).

2.8.2. d. Antipyretic medications:

Paracetamol remains the safest drug among all antipyretics and analgesic drugs, as its use for all patients with COVID-19 to reduce their temperature and relieve pain with very few side effects that are almost rare compared to other medicines. It can be used from the onset of symptoms until recovery (Sestili, & Fimognari, 2020).

2.8.2. e. Anticoagulant medications: Recent evidence points to the risk of arterial and venous thrombotic complications due to excessive inflammation, platelet activation, endothelial dysfunction and a high risk of thrombosis during acute infection with COVID-19. These cases can treated with oral anticoagulant agents as a (Rivaroxaban) or alternative parenteral anticoagulant drugs such as low molecular weight heparin (LMWH) (Di Tano, et al., 2020). Rivaroxaban is an oral anticoagulant agent. Its dose is 15 mg twice daily with food for 3 weeks, then 20 mg daily with food. The mode of action of rivaroxaban is a direct inhibitor of factor Xa. The primary mechanism of elimination of rivaroxaban is through the Kidney with a half-life of 5-9 hrs. Rivaroxaban is contraindication for active pathological bleeding and severe hypersensitivity (Rizk, et al., 2021).

2.8.2. f. Immune boosting against COVID-19:

Studies have indicated that COVID-19 affects the immune system by producing systemic infections response or cytokine release syndrome as well as influenced by it. It is well known that the elderly are the most affected by complications COVID-19 either directly or through several age-related comorbidities. Many studies have proven that good health comes through healthy nutrition that includes all nutritional components of salts, proteins, carbohydrates, fats, vitamins, and others. The most important immune-supporting nutrients are zinc, selenium, omega-3, fatty acids and vitamins C, D, and E (Shakoor, et al., 2021).

2.8.2.f.1. Vitamin D:

Vitamin D boosts innate immunity by increasing the expression of antimicrobial peptides including cathelicidin and defensins. Defensins boost the expression of anti-oxidant genes. Vitamin D is believed to help keep pulmonary tissues healthy. Low levels of vitamin D receptor expression result in increased claudin-2 expression and inflammation. Some studies indicate an inverse relationship between upper respiratory infection and serum levels of 25-hydroxyvitamin D. Supplementation may reduce pro-inflammation Cytokines and thus reduction of mortality associated with acute respiratory distress syndrome in COVID-19 patients (Gorman, 2017).

2.8.2.f.2. Vitamin C:

Vitamin C has been recommended as a counter to the cytokine storm that occurs after COVID-19 infection as the disease develops. Pro-inflammatory cytokines are known to be reduced by vitamin C, whereas anti-inflammatory cytokines are increased such as Interleukin 10 (IL-10). In COVID-19, IL-10 regulates inflammation by acting as a negative feedback mechanism with Interleukin 6 (IL-6). Vitamin C consumption of 1 gram per day has been shown in clinical trials to enhance IL-10 production (Shakoor, et al., 2021).

2.8.2.f.3. Zinc:

Zinc has the potential to be a supportive therapy in COVID-19 patients due to its immunomodulatory and antiviral characteristics. Zinc supplementation has been recommended as a way to improve the efficacy of other therapies presently being studied, such as hydroxychloroquine. A large dosage of zinc can help with clinical symptoms and can help with

COVID-19 related symptoms such as lower respiratory tract infection (Finzi, 2020).

2.8.2.f.4. Omega-3 and fatty acids:

Omega-3 and fatty acids, which comprise eicosapentaenoic and docosahexaenoic fatty acids, are polyunsaturated fatty acids that have been shown to improve immunity and inflammation. Omega-3 fatty acids, for example, have antiviral properties by decreasing influenza virus replication. The intake of omega-3 fatty acids may enhance oxygenation in COVID-19 patients (Rogero, et al., 2020).

2.9. Benefits of positioning for patient with COVID-19:

Positioning is a physiologic mechanism that helps patients with COVID-19 to improve oxygenation and decrease dyspnea. There are several useful positions for the patient, including the prone position which is when the patient lies on his face, abdomen and chest is close to the floor to improve oxygenation and decreased lung injury by reducing V/Q mismatch. But in this position expansion of the anterior chest wall is restricted. Since the prone position limits the movement of the rib cage, which negatively affects the expansion of the lungs (Venus, et al., 2020).

2.9.1. The effect of position on severity of dyspnea and cough:

Moghadam, et al., (2020) indicated that the prone position had a positive effect on 60% of patients regarding improved dyspnea and SpO_2 for all patients after applying this position. A study conducted by Baysal, et al., (2018) reported that the prone position and the tripod position had the same positive effect on the severity of dyspnea, and it was clear from the presence of statistical significance among them. While the supine position has a lesser effect than the previous two positions on the severity of dyspnea. Prone positioning and tripod position improve oxygenation and decreases the level of dyspnea because it shifts of fluid from the dorsal alveoli, allowing it to be recruited and filled with oxygenated air, thereby improve gas exchange, and lung ventilation.

2.9.2. The effect of position on cardiopulmonary parameters:

Baysal, et al., (2018) reported that tripod position gives the best subjective easing of SOB, reduce RR, and improve SpO_2 in patient with COPD patients. The prone and tripod position had the same positive effect on measurement of SBP, DBP, SpO_2, RR, and HR. During prone position, the heart falls away from the lung anteriorly and the left lower pulmonary vein. This position helps to a more favorable venous return to the heart, which might explain the improvement in hemodynamic parameters noted in patients (McNicholas, 2020). Sartini, et al., (2020) stated that all patients had improvement in PaO_2 and 80% of them had improvement of SpO_2 and all patients had decreased of RR after implementing prone position. A study done by Mahrous, & Aboelmagd, (2022) exposed that the knee-chest position significantly improved some cardiopulmonary indicators through reduced RR and PR and increased SpO_2 in preterm babies.

2.10. Benefits of coughing exercises on severity of dyspnea, cough, and cardiopulmonary parameters for patient with COVID-19:

There are several respiratory problems that associated with COVID-19 such as sticky secretions inside the bronchial tree that lead to inflammation or pulmonary fibrosis, which may be lead to acute respiratory failure. Coughing exercises should be applied for patients with COVID-19 that relieve pain, helps to get rid secretion, thereby improve lung ventilation and reduce dyspnea (Jarosz, et al., 2020). Nolt, et al., (2007) reported that acute cough causes abnormal changes in some cardiopulmonary parameters. It is emphases that 50% of patients had SpO_2 < 90%, 43.1% had RR was > 30 breath \ minute, and 42.7% had PR > 100 beats \ minute.

2.11. Theoretical framework: Core, Care, Cure model:

Introduction of theorist:

Lydia Hall was born on September 21st, 1906, in New York City. She graduated with a bachelor of science and a master of arts from Columbia University's Teacher's College after graduating from York Hospital School of Nursing in Pennsylvania. She died of heart disease in Queens Hospital in New York on February 27th, 1969. She would not classify herself as a nurse-theorist. She didn't set out to create a nursing theory; rather, she wanted to present a perspective on professional nursing (Alligood, 2017). Hall articulated her thoughts regarding the significance of professional nursing to patient wellbeing based on her observations of hospital treatment at the time. She was also opposed to the philosophy of team nursing, which was popular at the time in many acute care facilities (Alligood, 2014). Hall was confident that providing direct care by a professional nurse improves patient outcomes. Hall thought that the major focus should be on care, and that nurses were the most suited to give the type of care that would allow patients to reach their full potential (Priyadarshini, 2021).

The Focus on the Research and Interest:

- Hall developed the Care, Cure, Core theory after conducting research in the field of chronically ill patient rehabilitation.
- Hall was interested in rehabilitative nursing and the role that the professional nurse had in the patient's recovery and welfare
- Hall founded the Loeb Center for Nursing and Rehabilitation at Montefiore Medical Center in Bronx, New York, and served as its first director (Smith, 2010).

Aspects of Hall's theory:

Core: The third area that nursing shares with all of the helping professions is that of using relationships for therapeutic effect —the core. The patient is the center of the nursing process to achieve all his needs that include; physical, social, emotional, spiritual, and intellectual needs (Sumarno, 2019). The nurse gives explanations and treatment goals in the "core" aspect to aid in the process of improving patient awareness. Self-awareness allows a person to develop self-control (Umara, 2018).

Care: is what the nurse does to take care of the patient's body. The intent of bodily care is to comfort the patient (Sumarno, 2019). The job of nurses in health care is prevention or preventive and health care, according to Hall's theory (Umara, 2018).

Cure: It is the outcome or end result of the nursing care that is achieved the nurse helping of the patient through his or her medical, surgical, and rehabilitative care in the role of comforter (Sumarno, 2019). A form of cure was delivered to the patient in the method of therapy and medical care. In this instance, the nurse and the doctor work together to provide nursing care (Umara, 2018).

Meta-paradigm concept of Hall:

- **Person:** Hall believed that through this process, the patient would emerge as a whole person (Alligood, 2017
- **Health:** a state of self-awareness accompanied by the deliberate selection of behaviors that are most appropriate for that individual the requirement to assist the client in exploring the meaning of his or her behavior in order to recognize and solve difficulties through developing self-identity and maturity (Alligood, 2017).
- **Environment:** Hall considered that the hospital environment provides experience for the patient during treatment for acute disease (Smith, 2010).
- **Nursing**: Participation in the care, core, and cure aspects of the patient's care (Smith, 2010).

Assumptions:

- The patient's motivation and energy rather than the healthcare team's, are required for the cure.

- The core, care, cure aspects are interrelated and should not be viewed it as functioning independently.
- The three aspects interact, and the circles representing them change size, depending on the patient's total course of progress (Smith, 2010).

Lydia hall's theory application in the nursing process

- ❖ The core, care, cure theory will be applicable in an assessment, planning, and implementation of patient's care
- ❖ Establishing a nurse-patient relationship to improve the care that achieves the requirements of the patient with professional nursing care (Smith, 2010).

Practical application of theory:

Core: The non- intubated patient infected with COVID-19 suffers from several problems associated with COVID-19 infection, including dyspnea, cough, and cardiopulmonary parameters alterations.

Care: The nurse helped the patients to implement prostrate position for a full hour and to perform coughing exercises at the same time to treat problems that, including dyspnea, cough, and cardiopulmonary parameters alterations.

Cure: The nurse solved the patient's problems (dyspnea, cough, and cardiopulmonary parameters alterations) through the application of the interventional protocol (prostrate position and coughing exercises). Dyspnea was relieved, as well as coughing and cardiopulmonary parameters alterations were improved.

2.12. Previous related studies:

First Study:

A quasi-experimental study was conducted by Mahrous, and Aboelmagd, (2022), was carried out at the Neonatal Intensive Care Unit in Egypt. 57 preterm neonates with RDS include in the study in the non-probability method (purposive sample). To determine the effect of knee-chest position, semi-sitting, and right sideline position on preterm neonates with RDS. The results of this study found that the knee-chest position significantly improved some cardiopulmonary parameters such as increased PaO_2 and decreased RR and PR.

Second Study:

An experimental study was conducted by Ibraheem, et.al, (2021), on 52 COVID-19 patients in Tikrit City, from 1st June to 30th August 2020 to assess the application of prone positioning in management of a wake spontaneously breathing patients. The results of this study were indicated that the prone position helps relieve SOB and increase the level of SpO_2 among patients with COVID-19. Thus it will help to reduce the need for ventilators and will reduce the death rate due to hypoxia among COVID-19 patients.

Third Study:

Quazi- experimental study was conducted by Arık, & Çevik, (2021). This include 100 patients who diagnosed with COPD, between November 2016 and April 2017, in the state hospital in Turkey. Postural drainage and deep breathing-coughing exercises were performed twice a day, morning and evening for 7 days. Hemodynamic parameters were recorded four times a day, pre-exercise and post-exercise. The forced vital capacity (FVC), forced expiratory volume (FEV1) and FEV1 / FVC values obtained during the pulmonary function test (PFT) were assessed at the end of the first day of the study before the exercise and at the end of the 7th day to examine the effect of postural drainage and deep breathing-cough exercises on oxygen saturation, and lung function in COPD patients. It was reported that there was a statistically significant difference in the oxygen saturation, triflo volume, and PFT of the patients on all days before and after exercise.

Fourth Study:

A study was done by Langer, et al., (2021), a multi-centric study for more than 1000 patients. This study conducted in Italy on adult patients requiring invasive mechanical ventilation for respiratory failure caused by COVID-19 were studied retrospectively in 24 Italian Intensive Care Units (ICU) between February 24th and June 14th, 2020. On the day of ICU admission, clinical data were obtained. Every day, data on the utilization of the prone posture was gathered. On July 15th, 2020, patient outcomes were followed upon. In a subgroup of 78 individuals, the respiratory consequences of the initial prone position were investigated. Patients were labeled as oxygen responders if their fraction of inspired oxygen PaO_2/FiO_2 ratio increased by more than 20 mmHg when prone, and as carbon dioxide responders if their ventilator ratio increased by more than 20 mmHg. The results of this study were mild, moderate, and severe ARDS were observed in 15%, 50%, and 35 % of the patients, respectively, with death rates of 25%, 33%, and 41%. In 61 percent of the patients, the prone position was used. Overall, prone position increased $PaO_2 \backslash FiO_2$ ratios significantly.

Fifth Study:

Altinay, et al., (2021) conducted a study in turkey from March 15th to June 15th, 2020 of 24 Patients with COVID-19 who admitted into ICU, prone position applied on them. The result of study exposed that median of SpO_2 before prone positioning was 89% but, after positioning 95%, median of PaO_2 was 65 mm hg and become 82 mm Hg, also the median of $PaCO_2$ change from 36 mm Hg to 30 mm Hg.

Sixth Study:

Moghadam, et al., (2020) done a study on 10 COVID-19 patients in Iran, the sample was chosen randomly to identify role of prone positioning in the management of COVID-19, reported that the patients were males with a percentage of 70% and 30% are females. Not all of them had endotracheal intubation; none of them used mechanical respiration. The mean age of the patients was 41 years, 30% of them have a previous medical history with hypertension or diabetes. After applying the prone position to the patients, the mean of SpO_2 was 85.6% and 95.9%. The feeling of decreased dyspnea for 40% of cases and all patients were likewise he got out of the hospital. The median duration of hospitalization for these patients was 4.8 days and no deaths.

Seventh Study:

Thompson, et al. (2020) conducted a study on 88 consecutive patients admitted to the Columbia University step-down unit (intermediate care unit) between April 6th and April 14th, 2020. Inclusion criteria were laboratory-confirmed COVID-19 with severe hypoxemia. Results among 29 eligible patients, 25 had at least one awake session of the prone position lasting longer than 1 hour; 4 refused the prone position and were intubated immediately .One hour after initiation of the prone position, SpO_2 increased compared with baseline. The range of improvement in SpO_2 was 1% to 34%. Among all patients, the levels of supplemental oxygen were unchanged during the first hour of the prone position. One hour after initiation of the prone position, 19 patients had SpO_2 of 95% or greater.

Eight Study:

Zang, et al., (2020) conducted a study in china, which a single-center prospective cohort study the study was from February 1st, 2020, to April 30th, 2020, a total of 60 COVID-19 patients with severe hypoxia were enrolled. In addition, 23 patients were placed in the early prone position, whereas 37 were not. Reported that the SpO_2 in the prone position group increased from 91.09,or 1.54 % to 95.30, or 1.72 % after 10 minutes, 95.48, or 1.73 % after 30 minutes, but there was no significant difference after 30 minutes compared to 10 minutes. After 10 minutes, the RR decreased from 28.22, (3.06 times/min) to 27.78, (2.75 times/min), and from 24.87, (1.84 times/min) to 24.87, (1.84 times/min) after 30 minutes.

Ninth Study:

A study conducted in New York by Damarla, et al., (2020), from March 23th, 2020, to April 15th, 2020, A total of 10 COVID-19 patients enrolled in the study were placed in a prone position for two hours to identify the effect of this position on RR and SpO_2. The results of the study exposed that 30% of the patients were female and 70% were males, and the median age was 56 years, 70% of the patients did not require intensive respiratory care and 80% of the patients did not require intubation.

Literature synthesis:

Previous studies indicated that most COVID-19 patients were elderly, male, and suffering from several problems associated with this disease, including dyspnea, a decrease in SpO_2, a decrease in PaO_2, breadypnea, increase of $PaCo_2$, hypertension, tachycardia, in addition to a persistent cough. The researchers tried several interventions to reduce the problems mentioned above, these interventions including prone position, deep breathing exercises, and coughing exercises. These studies concluded that the above interventions were able to increase SpO_2 and PaO_2. It was also able to reduce the severity of dyspnea, cough, RR, PR, $PaCo_2$, the need for ventilation, and the hospitalization periods. In addition to that there was a study that conducted on preterm neonates with RDS to find out the effect of the different positions, including knee-chest, semi-sitting, and right sideline. It reported that the knee-chest position considerably improved various cardiopulmonary measures, such as increased PaO_2 and lowered RR and PR.

Chapter three

Methods

&

Procedures

Chapter three

Methods and Procedures

This chapter will present all the methodological procedures that were applied in this study in detail for the purpose of achieving the set goals. These procedures were including the design of the study, administrative arrangements, ethical consideration, settings of the study, method of sample selecting, steps of the study, inclusion / exclusion criteria, instrumentation, methods of data collection, and data analysis.

3.1. Design of the study:

An experimental study design by which a patient infected with COVID-19 virus manage within a prostrate position, and coughing exercises, and then measuring their effect on the severity of cough and dyspnea level, as well as their effect on cardiopulmonary parameters. The study was conducted at Imam Hussain Medical City/COVID-19 wards in Holy Kerbala city; the period of the study was from 25th October, 2021 to 1st May, 2022.

3.2. Administrative arrangements:

Formal administrative approvals to conduct the study were obtained from the following institutions prior to actual data collection:

a. University of Kerbala / Collage of Nursing (Appendix AI).
b. Ministry of Health / Kerbala Health Department / Imam Hussain Medical City (Appendix AII).
c. Ministry of Health / Kerbala Health Department / Training and Human Development Center (Appendix AIII).

3.3. Ethical consideration:

The research ethics committee at the University of Kerbala /College of nursing provided ethical permission for the secrecy and anonymity of the participants' identities as shown in Appendices B. The participants were thoroughly informed of the present study and its objectives, and it was made clear to them that they had the right to withdraw from the study at any moment, thus they gave their voluntarily oral and written agreement to participate in this study. In addition to that, the researcher considered the confidentiality of the gathered data as shown Appendix K.

3.4. Settings of the Study:

This study was conducted in the COVID-19 wards in Imam Hussein Medical City in Kerbala. Imam Hussein Medical City is the largest health institution in the Kerbala city, which contains surgical, medical, and infectious diseases wards, contains 600 beds for inpatients. After the outbreak of the COVID-19 pandemic in the Kerbala governorate, approximately 200 beds were allocated to receive COVID-19 patients, including 12 beds for critical cases.

3.5. Sample size:

The selected sample size was 60 patients divided into two groups. There were 30 patients for each control and experiment groups. The sample was selected by systematic random sampling method. A list was arranged for all members' inclusion population. The process involved choosing each individual to list, using a randomly selected starting point that was number two. The number and size of elements in the population were determined by the required sample. Then the researcher divided the population size by the desired sample size, giving k^{th}, the size of the gap between the selected elements from the list. The access population size was $N = 131$ and the required sample size is $n = 60$, the value of kth will be: according to the following equation $K^{th} = 131 \div 60 = 2.1 \approx 2$. Thus, $k^{th} = 2$, which means that every 2 person on the list was included in the sample. To prevent the occurrence of any bias during the selection of the sample and to give strength to the research, the researcher excludes himself from selecting the elements of the sample and assigning the task of selection to another person (Gray, et al., 2016).

3.6. Sample of the study:

A probability (Systematic random) sampling was selected from non-intubated patients with COVID-19 who were hospitalized in COVID-19 wards at Imam Hussein Medical City in Holy Kerbala. 30 patients were enrolled as a control group and 30 patients were enrolled as a study group. The study group participants were exposed to an interfering protocol (applying prostrate position for full one hour and make coughing exercises as the same time). The selection criteria were established as follow:

3.6.1. Inclusion Criteria: shown in figure (3-1)

- A hospitalized patient who were already diagnosed with COVID-19 who had a lung CT scan.
- Both male and female gender.
- Those who were non-intubated.
- Those who had cough and dyspnea.
- Patients who are willing to participate in the study.
- Patients who intellectually competent and able to communicate verbally.

3.6.2. Exclusion Criteria:

The researcher excluded all of the following as shown in figure (3-1)

- Pilot study participants.
- Patients with COVID-19 who do not have a cough.
- Patients with COVID-19 who do not have a dyspnea.
- Patients with COVID-19 who are refused to participate in the study.
- Patients with COVID-19 who do not have a lung CT scan.

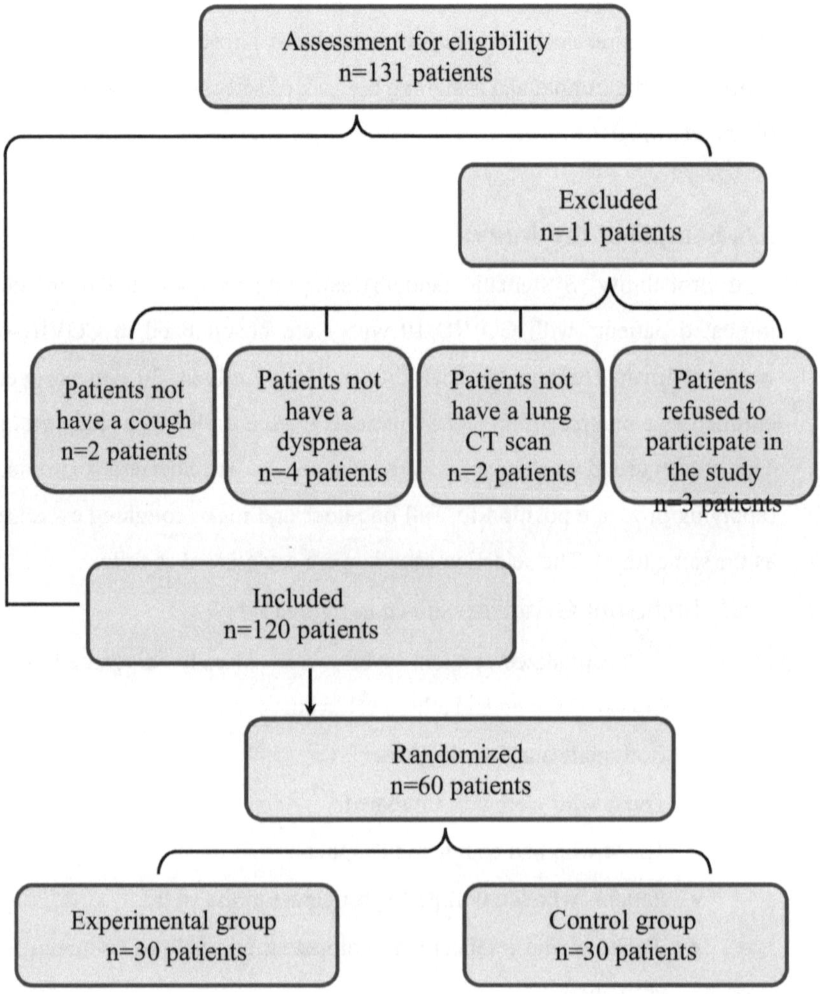

Figure (3-1): Flowchart of the randomized control trial & eligibility criteria

3.7. Steps of the Study:

The present study is conducted according to the following steps:

3.7.1. Interventional protocol:

The interventional protocol was design based on information gained from a review of the comparative scientific literature and previous studies, as well as the researcher's experience in caring for patients with COVID-19 and based on their needs to reduce the disease's consequences. This protocol is designed to include how to take the prostrate position and its times, as well as how to do coughing exercises during this position. The interventional protocol consists of two overlapping procedures (prostrate position and coughing exercises) so that the patient is placed in prostrate position for a full hour and the coughing exercises are performed for the patient at the first time of prostration.

a- Prostrate position:

The patient lies down so that his knees, forehead, and hands are close to the ground and the elbows are flexed and relaxed to bear the weight of the patient as shown in the Appendices CI, and CII. The abdominal area remains unsupported so that the position of the patient is the same as the position of prostrate during prayer.

b- Coughing exercises:

Coughing exercises are performed during the first minutes of the hour designated for prostrate position. It is achieved by performing the following steps:

- Percuss on the upper back (in the field of the lung) to move the sticky secretions from inside the alveoli to the bronchioles to facilitate their expulsion as shown in appendix CIII.
- Ask the client to take two or three deep breaths slowly through the nose and exhale through the mouth.

- Instruct client to inhale deeply, hold breath for several seconds and cough twice while exhaling. The first cough loosens the mucus; the second expels secretions.
- Ask client to exhale sharply with a "huff" sound mid-exhalation. This technique helps keep your airways open while moving secretions up and out of the lungs.
- Rest and breathe slowly between coughs.
- Try to avoid prolonged episodes of coughing because these may cause fatigue and hypoxia.
- This exercise is stopped as soon as the patient feels secretions running out or feels comfortable (Berman, et al., 2016).

This interventional protocol (prostrate position and coughing exercises) allows lung secretions to exit and helps the patient to get rid of them as well as helps the lungs to fully expansion thereby reducing dyspnea, relief cough, and correction the cardiopulmonary alterations as shown figures (3-2) and (3-3).

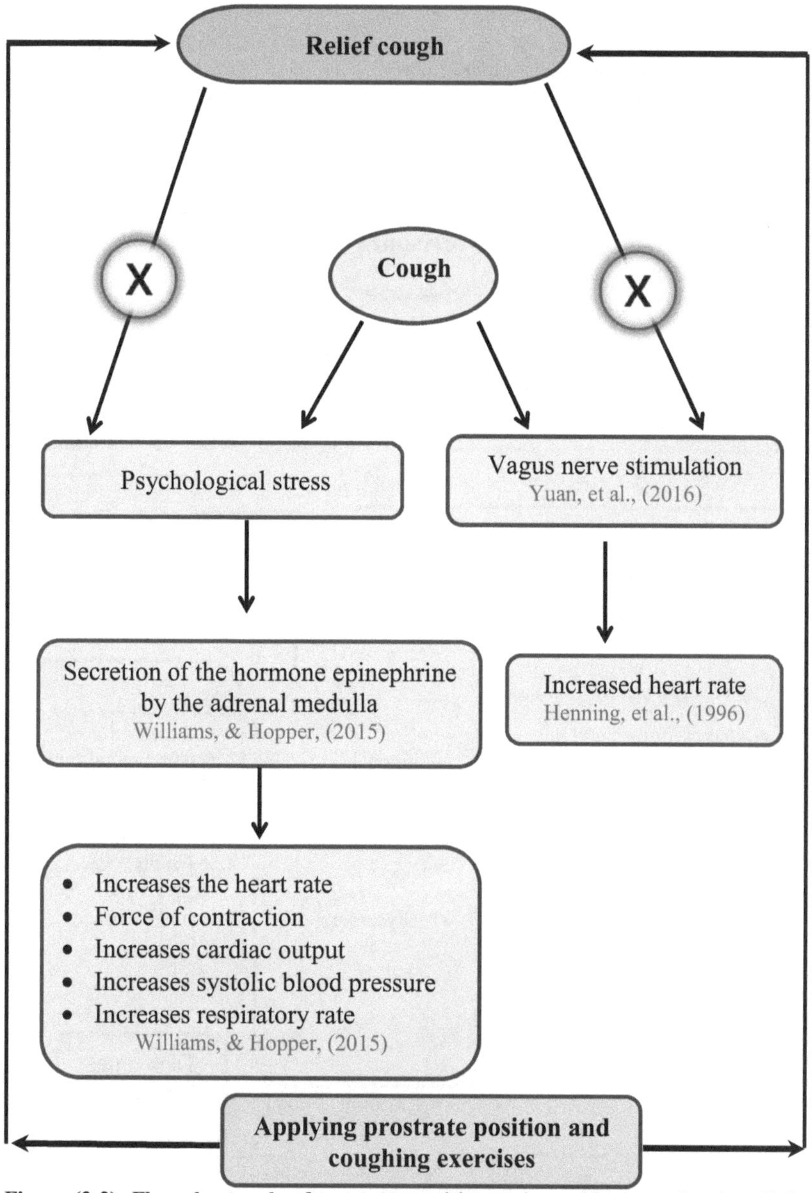

Figure (3-2): Flow chart: role of prostrate position and coughing exercises in relief cough and improving cardiopulmonary parameters.

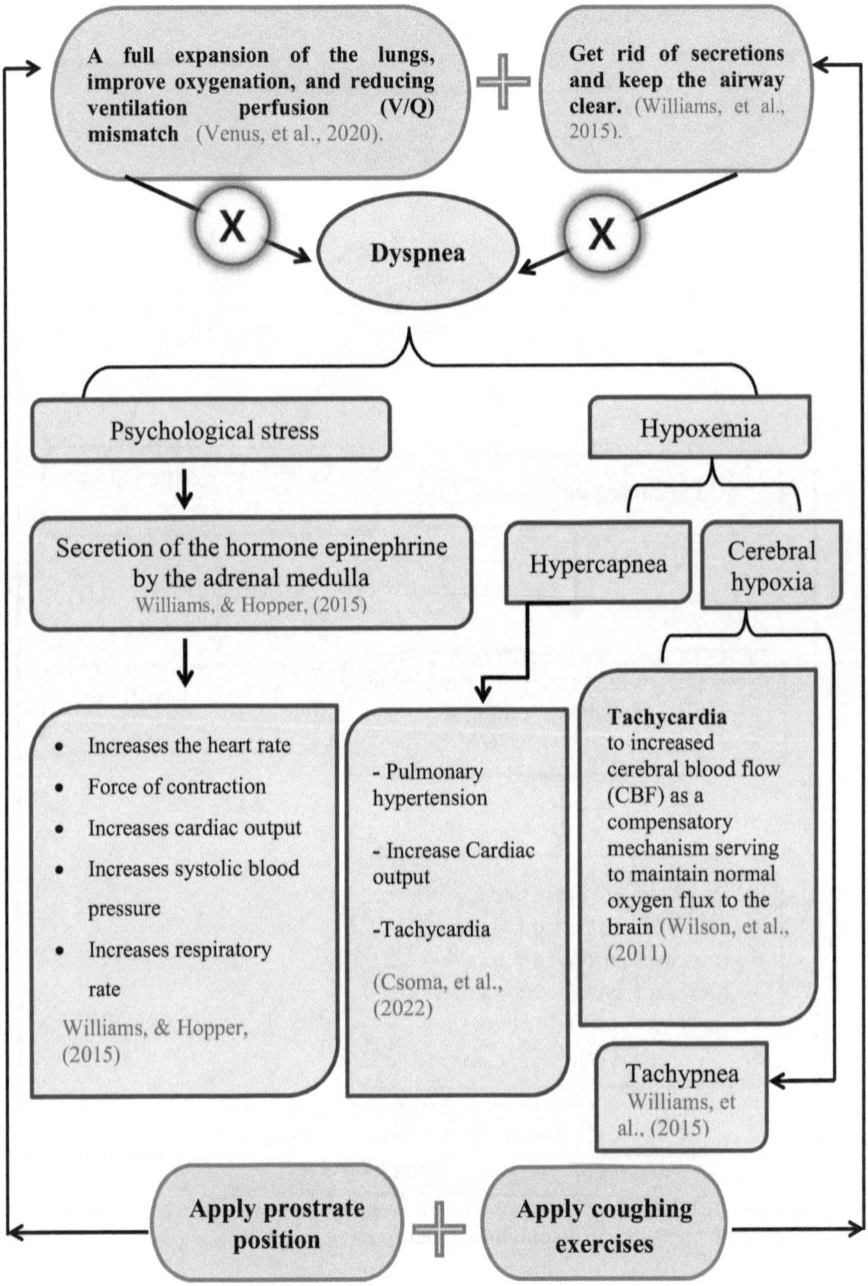

Figure (3-3): Flow chart: role of prostrate position and coughing exercises in relief dyspnea and improving cardiopulmonary parameters.

3.7.2. The study instruments:

To achieve the objectives of the study, a questionnaire format is designed and modifying after review the related the literature and the previous studies. The instruments consists from four parts.

Part (1) Socio-demographic and clinical data questioner: this part includes age, gender, smoking status, second hand smoke, body mass index, chronic diseases, chronic medications use, medications currently use (bronchodilators, antipyretics, and antitussive, infected part of the lung, percentage of infected area, duration from first symptom appearance, duration of hospitalization, oxygen therapy status, and COVID-19 vaccination as shown in the appendix DI.

Part (2) cardiopulmonary parameters chart: As shown in appendix DII this part includes SBP and DBP which measured by sphygmomanometer , PP that measured through applying the following formula (PP= SBP-DBP), PR and SpO_2 measured by pulse oximetry device , RR was calculated by observing and calculating the number of times the patient's chest rise and fall during one minute, CO was measured by applying the following formula (CO=(PPxHR)*2ml) (Koenig, et al., 2015), While the MAP is measured by applying the formula of (MAP = ([DBP x 2] + SBP) ÷ 3 (Farrell, & Dempsey, 2010).

Part (3) Dyspnea index (DI): This index consist of 10 items designed by Gartner-Schmidt, et al., (2014), as shown in appendix J to measure the level of dyspnea. This scale has been modified in response to expert opinions to be suitable for measuring the phenomenon under study as shown in appendix DIII, after the approval was obtained for its use as indicated in appendix H.

Part (4) Cough severity index (CSI): This index contain 10 items, it is a scale that has been modified in response to the opinions of experts to be suitable for measuring the phenomenon under study as shown in appendix DIV to measure the severity of a patient's cough. The original scale was designed by Shembel, et al., (2013) as shown in appendix I. The approval was obtained for its use as indicated in appendix H.

3.8. Testing the Validity and Reliability for instrumentation:

3.8.1. Study Instrument Validation:

The instrument validation .indicates an extent to that it actual reflection or an able for measuring the phenomena which need examined the validation process is a truths of a research Validation of an experimental researches representing an extent to which the research examines it's under the hypothesis, that allow the support to the level of concept of research, its theoretical framework (Gray, et al., 2016). The interventional protocol and the study instrument (appendices DI-DIV) underwent series of revisions and modifications according to panel (19) experts as shown in appendix E, those experts had more than ten years of experience in their field of specialty. The researcher proposed each expert member to review the study instrument for content, simplicity, relevance, style, and suitability.

3.8.1.1. The content validation:

Yusoff, (2019) define it as "the degree to which elements of an assessment instrument are relevant to and representative of the targeted construct for a particular assessment purpose" Both cough severity index (CSI) and dyspnea index (DI) scale translate to Arabic language by back Brisilin's back translation model. Researcher did content validation and content validity index depend on (Yusoff, 2019). Thought apply content validation process:

1) Preparing the validation form to the review panel of the experts that will had the understanding about the process and the clear expectations.
2) The researcher distributed questioner to (7) review panel of experts that are have more than 10 years of professional experience in the field of specialty, these experts are (4) members from college of

nursing - University of Baghdad, (1) member from the college of nursing - University of Babylon, (1) member from the college of nursing -University of Kufa, (1) member from the college of nursing -University of Kirkuk. Content validity conducted by face to face through researcher meeting with experts and by non-face to face by sent form to experts online.

3) Reviewing items are clearly provided to the experts and they provided score on each item also comment on some items and all comment the researcher taken in consideration.
4) The scores provided through the experts on each the item independent based on relevant scales.
5) Finally, calculate the content validation index (CVI) as follow:

a) **Cough severity index (CSI)**: Number of experts was (7). experts in agreement for each question was (7,7,7,6,7,6,7,7,6,7). Universal agreement (UA) for each item was (1, 1, 1, 0, 1, 0, 1, 1, 0, and 1). I- CVR (item level content validity index) for each item was (1, 1, 1, 0.7, 1, 0.7, 1, 1, 0.7, and 1). S-CVI\Ave (the scales\levels of content validation index based on an average method) of this scale was (0.91) and this value acceptable for CVI (Yusoff, 2019). Yusoff, (2019) explain the term of S-CVI\UA as "scale-level content validity index based on the universal agreement .method". It was (0.7) the Average of proportions of all items were judged as relevant across 7 experts were (0.91) as shown in the appendix FI.

b) **Dyspnea index (DI):** Number of experts was (7). Experts in agreement for each question was (7,6,7,7,7,7,7,7,6, 6). Universal agreement (UA) for each item was (1, 0, 1, 1, 1, 1, 1, 1, 0, and 0). I- CVI (item level content validity index) for each item was (1, 0.7, 1, 1, 1, 1, 1, 1, 0.7, and 0.7). S-CVI\Ave of this scale was (0.91) and this value acceptable for CVI (Yusoff, 2019). S-CVI\UA was (0.7). The Average of proportions of all items were judged as relevant across 7 experts were (0.95) as shown in the appendix FII.

3.8.1.2. Face validity:

Yusoff, (2019) knows it as "the responses the process of the validation were refer to the degree to which test .respondents view the content of a test and its items as relevant to the context in which the test is being administered commonly, response process validity evidence is performed after content validity has been established".

The following are the six steps of response process validation:

1) The first step it was preparing responses steps of validity form to that the raters, who had an understanding for this process and the clear expectations .
2) The researcher distributed questioner to (12) review panel of experts are have 10 years of professional experience in their fields or more, these experts are (4) from faculty member of college of nursing \University of Baghdad, (2) from faculty member of college of nursing \University of Kerbala, (5) from Kerbala Health Department / Imam Hussain Medical City, and (1) A member of the College of Nursing - University of Warith Al-Anbiya.
3) The process of response validity done by face, to, face or by the online assessment method.
4) In this step, domain of items were sent to panel of the raters reviewers were asked to review these items before submitting the score for these items. Reviewers are encouraged for providing a written his commitments for improving an understanding and the clarity of each item.

5) After complete of review each item, the reviewers asked for providing the scores for all items. The researcher received scores responses from the reviewers.
6) There were 2 forms of FVI, (I-.FVI) for the items and S-FVI for the scale and items. Proportion of scale that complete comprehension scales and a clarity of three or four by all reviewers (S-FVI/UA) In this last step the face Viability Index (FVI) was calculated :

a) **Cough severity index (CSI)**: Number of raters was (12) Raters in agreement for each question were (10, 12, 10, 9, 12, 12, 10, 12, 12, and 12). Universal agreement (UA) for each item was (0, 1, 0, 0, 1, 1, 0, 1, 1, and 1). I- FVI (item face validity index) for each item was (0.83, 1, 0.83, 0.75, 1, 1, 0.83, 1, 1, and1). S-CVI\Ave .of this scale was (0.92) and this value acceptable for FVI (Yusoff, 2019). S-FVI\UA was (0.7). Proportion average of the items judgment as comprehension and the clarity across the seven experts was (0.91) as shown in the appendices GI.

b) **Dyspnea index (DI)**: Number of raters was (12). Raters in agreement for each question were (11, 12, 11, 12, 12, 12, 12, 12, 12, and 11). Universal agreement (UA) for each item was (0, 1, 0, 1, 1, 1, 1, 1, 1, and 0). I- FVI (item of face validation index) for each item was (0.9, 1, 0.9, 1, 1, 1, 1, 1, 1, and 0.9). S-CVI\Ave (scale-face validity index based on .the average method) of this scale was (0.95) and this value .acceptable for FVI (Yusoff, 2019). S-FVI\UA was (0.7). Average proportion of items judged as clarity and comprehension across the seven experts was (0.96) as shown in the appendix GII.

c) **3.8.2. Pilot Study**:

A pilot study was conducted at AL-Husain Medical City in Kerbala City. It was carried out on (10) patients who had the same criteria of the study sample in the period from December 2nd 2021 to December 14th 2021. It was collected by systematic random sampling method. The sample of pilot study was excluded from the original sample of the study.

3.8.2.1. Pilot studypurposes:

a) To examines the reliability of the questionnaire.

b) To test the feasibility to answer the questionnaire.

c) To detect the total time required for each participants.

3.8.2.2. Pilot study results:

1. The questionnaires were clear.
2. The time needed to fill out the socio-demographic and clinical data part and two scales (CSI & DI) was 10-15 minutes.
3. The time required to check cardiopulmonary parameters was 10-15 minutes.
4. The total time that was sufficient to complete all data related to the questionnaire at each time ranged between 20-30 minutes.
5. The time required for data collecting from the patient from the first measurement of data (before implementing the intervention) to the fourth data measurement (seven hours after the end of the intervention) was seven hours.

3.8.3. Reliability of the questionnaire format items:

Munro, (2005) define the reliability as " reliable the .of the questionnaire was used to determine the accuracy of the questionnaire, since the results showed very high level of stability and internal consistency of principle parts concerning item's responses' of the questionnaire" by using alpha Cronbach we calculate a major statistical parameter. The acceptable of reliability coefficients of the studied questionnaire concerning internal consistency (.Alpha Cronbach) is 0.70 as shows in the table of (3-1) by calculating the results which the questionnaire was meaningful , successfully, as well as designed questionnaire was reliable to the research phenomenon of (effect of prostrate position and coughing exercises upon level of dyspnea, persistent cough, and cardiopulmonary parameters among non-intubated patient with COVID-19) on the same population at any time in the future under assumption of stability of conditions on the studied population, and that are accounted on measuring improvements due to applying the suggested of interventional protocol.

Table (3-1): Reliable coefficient of researched questionnaire concerning internal consistency (Alpha Cronbach)

Reliable coefficient of researching questionnaire	Alpha (Cronbach - α)	Standard lower value	Assessment
Cough severity index (CSI)	0.86	0.70	Verified
Dyspnea index (DI)	0.90	0.70	Verified

3.9. Data Collection:

The data collection process was carried out through the interview technique, and the researcher measured the cardiopulmonary parameters by himself and recorded them in the study instrument. The data were collected for study sample in the period from December 27th 2021 to February 15th 2022. The data were collected through four times as shown the figure (3-2).

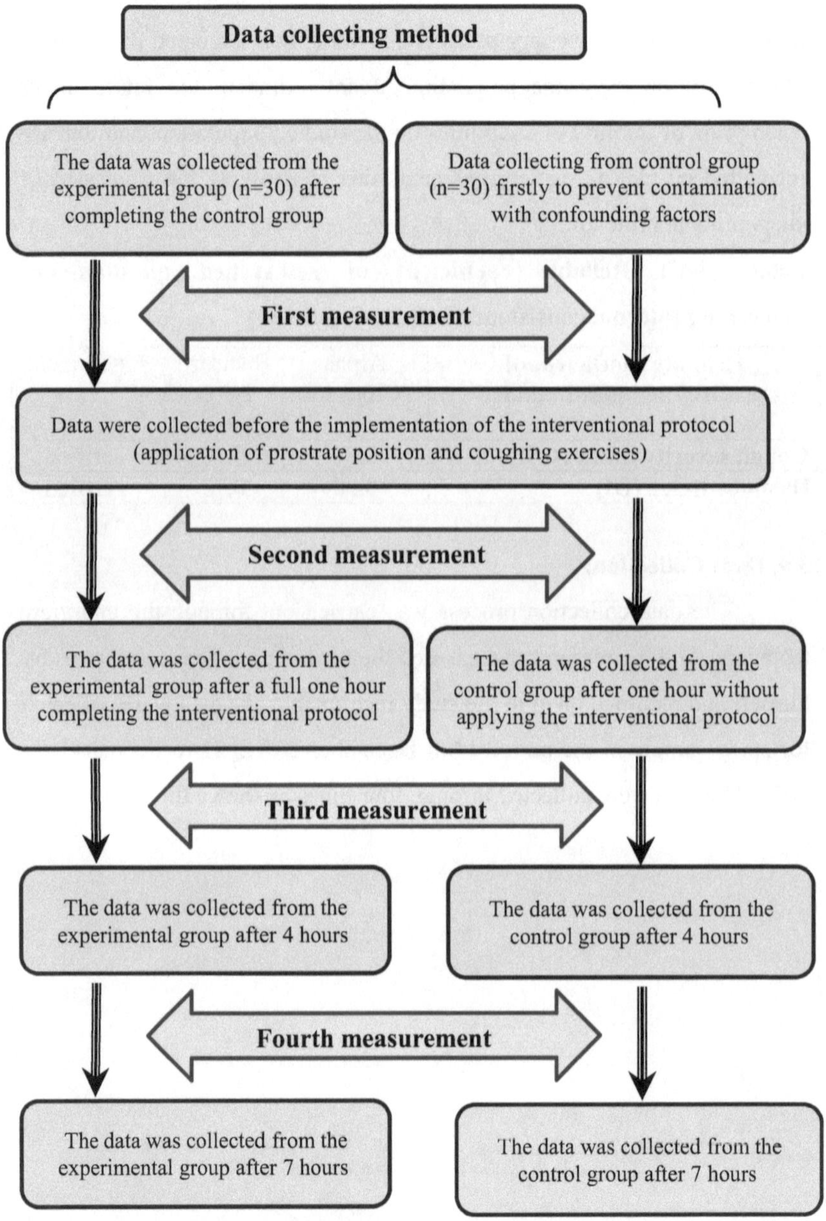

Figure (3-4): Flowchart of the data collecting method

3.10. Limitations:

There are a few significant limits to consider.

1- Most of the patients admitted to the hospital were critical and severe cases because patients with moderate or mild conditions refuse to be hospitalized and prefer to receive treatment at home.

2- Because the research is unique and original, we suffered from a lack of references.

3- There are several cardiopulmonary parameters such as PaO_2, $PaCO_2$, PH, HCO_3, and FIO_2 that have not been studied due to the lack of facilities.

3.11. Rating and scoring:

The items have been rated and scored according to the following patterns:

3.11.1. Rating and scoring for body mass index (BMI):

Body mass index was measured by measuring weight and height and applying the following formula:

BMI = weight in kilograms / (height in meters)^2 .Whereas BMI was categorized according to Hughes, (2022). As following data: underweight= less than 18.5, Normal body weight between18.5–24.9, while overweight about 25.0–29.9, obesity classified I between 30.0–34.9, obesity classified II= about 35.0–39.9, classified III more than 40 kg.

3.11.2. Rating and scoring for level of dyspnea and cough:

The dyspnea index respondent and cough severity index were scored with (2) for yes, (1) for no. The cutoff point was (1.5), the cutoff point is a critical value that represents the place in a theoretical distribution at which all attained values from the study sample that are equal to or beyond that point are assumed to be statistically significant (Nieswiadomy, 2012). The Cutoff point was calculated according to the following formula:

Cutoff point = (2+1)/ 2= 1.5, thereby the level of dyspnea is classified as follow:

Mild dyspnea = 1– 1.33, Moderate dyspnea = 1.34 – 1. 67, Sever dyspnea = 1. 68– 2.

And the level of cough is classified as follow:

Mild cough = 1– 1.33, Moderate cough = 1.34 – 1. 67, Sever cough = 1. 68– 2.

3.12. Statistical Data Analysis:

The data were analyzed by using the program of SPSS Version 25. Both descriptive and inferential statistical analysis approaches used in order to analyze and assess the study results, which are as follows:

3.12.1. Descriptive statistical Data Analysis:

Include percentage , mean, and frequency. The percentage (%) was calculated according to the following formula:

$$\% = \frac{\text{Frequencies}}{\text{Sample size}} \times 100$$

3.12.2. Inferential statistical Data Analysis:

- The analysis of variance (ANOVA) statistic (repeated-measures analysis of variance) is a parametric test that lets researchers to evaluate if the means of three or more measurements of the same person are similar or different.
- Chi-Square was used as a statistical method to measure the associations between the independent variables and the effect of the interventional protocol.
- The level of significance: It is well-defined as the probability value of rejecting a null hypothesis when it is true (Nieswiadomy, 2012). A probability value of ≤0.05 was considered statistically significant (Abd El Aziz, et al., 2016). Al-Kerety (2017) reported that the accepted probability value for significance was set to be <0.05% to >

0.01% indicating statistically significant, and $\leq$ 0.01% indicating highly significant statistical results.

Chapter four

Results & Findings

Chapter Four

Results and Findings

This chapter presents the results of the data analysis that are in correspondence with the early presented objectives. These results organized as follows:

Table (4-1): Distribution of participants according to their socio-demographic characteristics:

Socio-demographic Characteristics		Control group		Experimental group	
		f.	%	f.	%
Age (Per years)	< 40	2	6.7	3	10
	40 - < 60	8	26.7	8	26.7
	≥ 60	20	66.6	19	63.3
	Total	30	100	30	100
Gender	Male	14	46.7	18	60
	Female	16	53.3	12	40
	Total	30	100	30	100
Smoking condition	Never	20	66.7	23	76.7
	Previously	9	30	4	13.3
	Currently	1	3.3	3	10
	Total	30	100	30	100
Second-hand smoke	Yes	23	76.7	24	80
	No	7	23.3	6	20
	Total	30	100	30	100

f. (frequency); % (percentage)

Table (4-1) indicates that about two-thirds of the patients participating in the experimental and control groups are within the age groups of ≥ 60 years old and accounted for 63.3% for the experimental group, and 66.6% for the control group. 60% of the experimental group and 46.7% of the control group are males. While the greater percentage (76.7%) and (66.7%) of the patients who participated in the experimental and control groups respectively are never smoking. Furthermore, the majority of the experimental group exposed to second-hand smoke as well as more than three-quadrants of the control group also exposed to it.

***Table (4-2): Distribution of participants according to their* BMI:**

Body mass index	Control group		Experimental group	
	f.	%	f.	%
Normal weight	5	16.7	7	23.3
Overweight	7	23.3	1	3.3
Obesity class I	14	46.7	16	53.3
Obesity class II	3	10	3	10
Obesity class III	1	3.3	3	10
Total	30	100	30	100

f. (frequency); % (percentage)

This table shows that approximately half (46.7%) and (53.3%) of the patient participant in the experimental and control groups respectively were classified as obesity class I.

Table (4-3): Distribution of participants according to their clinical data:

Clinical data			Control group		Experimental group	
			f.	%	f.	%
Chronic diseases		Non	11	36.7	11	36.7
		Hypertension	7	23.3	4	13.3
		Asthma	9	30.0	8	26.7
		DM	3	10	7	23.3
		Total	30	100	30	100
Current medications use	Antitussive medications	Yes	28	93.3	28	93.3
		No	2	6.7	2	6.7
		Total	30	100	30	100
	Bronchodilator medications	Yes	10	33.3	9	30
		No	20	66.7	21	70
		Total	30	100	30	100
	Steroid medications	Yes	30	100	30	100
		No	0	0	0	0
		Total	30	100	30	100
	Antipyretic medications	Yes	26	86.7	28	93.3
		No	4	13.3	2	6.7
		Total	30	100	30	100

		f.	%	f.	%
Infected part of the lung	Bilateral-peripheral and central	12	40	13	43.3
	Bilateral central	8	26.7	12	40
	Bilateral peripheral	7	23.4	4	13.4
	Left lung- peripheral	1	3.3	1	3.3
	Right lung central	1	3.3	0	0
	Bilateral - lateral	1	3.3	0	0
	Total	30	100	30	100
Percent of the affected area	15 - 24%	5	16.7	0	0
	25 - 34%	5	16.7	3	10
	35 - 44%	5	16.7	3	10
	≥ 45 %	15	50	24	80
	Total	30	100	30	100
The period since the first appearance of symptoms (day)	1 - 3	1	3.3	2	6.7
	4 - 6	13	43.3	6	20
	≥ 7	16	53.4	22	73.3
	Total	30	100	30	100
Hospitalization period (day)	1 - 3	14	46.7	12	40
	4 - 6	15	50	14	46.7
	≥ 7	1	3.3	4	13.3
	Total	30	100	30	100
Method of oxygenation therapy	Face mask	20	66.7	18	60
	Re-breath mask	10	33.3	12	40
	Total	30	100	30	100
COVID-19 Vaccination	Yes	3	10	1	3.3
	No	27	90	29	96.7
	Total	30	100	30	100

f. (frequency); % (percentage)

Regarding the preexisting chronic diseases, as shown in table (4-3) the result exposed that 36.7% of both experimental and control groups did not have any chronic diseases. While 26.7% and 30% of the experimental and control groups respectively had asthma. Concerning to current medications use, about 93.3% of both experimental and control groups were treated with antitussive medications and 30% of the experimental group were treated with bronchodilators and 33.3% of the control group as well. As for steroid medications, all patients of both groups were treated with these medications. 93.3% of the experimental group was treated with antipyretics, as well as 86.7% of the control group. With regard to the infected part of the lung, 43.3% of the experimental group had bilateral-peripheral and central parts of the lung are infected, and 40% of the control group was also infected. Most of the patients had an infection rate of ≥ 45%, which was 80% of the experimental group and 50% of the control group. Furthermore, 73.3% of the experimental group and 53.4% of the control group had a period since the first appearance of symptoms was ≥ 7 days. The hospitalization period of most patients was 4-6 days, the percent for the experimental and control groups was 46.7% and 50%, respectively. The method of O_2 therapy for most patients was through a face mask, which accounted 60% of the experimental group, and 66.7% of the control group. Finally, 96.7% of the experimental group and 90% of the control group did not take the COVID-19 vaccine.

Table (4-4): Distributions of dyspnea and cough levels for the experimental and control groups

Variables		Experimental group								Control group							
		Before		After 1		After 2		After 3		Before		After 1		After 2		After 3	
		f.	%	f.	%	f.	%	f.	%	f.	%	f.	%	f.	%	f.	%
Level of Dyspnea	Mild	3	10	23	76.7	12	40	2	6.7	2	6.7	2	6.7	3	10	4	13.3
	Moderate	5	16.7	3	10	14	46.7	4	13.3	6	20	3	10	3	10	8	26.7
	Sever	22	73.3	4	13.3	4	13.3	24	80	22	73.3	25	83.3	24	80	18	60
	Total	30	100	30	100	30	100	30	100	30	100	30	100	30	100	30	100
Severity of Cough	Mild	3	10	19	63.4	17	56.7	5	16.7	3	10	2	6.7	2	6.7	3	10
	Moderate	5	16.7	7	32.3	11	36.6	8	26.7	7	32.3	1	3.3	3	10	3	10
	Sever	22	73.3	4	13.3	2	6.7	17	56.7	20	66.7	27	90	25	83.3	24	80
	Total	30	100	30	100	30	100	30	100	30	100	30	100	30	100	30	100

f: frequency; %: percentage; Before: before implementing the intervention; After 1: one hour after implement intervention, After 2: four hours after implement intervention; After 3: seven hours after implement intervention.

Table (4-4) shows the different levels of dyspnea and the cough between the experimental and control groups at the four measurements periods. As shown in the experimental group the level of dyspnea was as follows: 10% of patients were mild, 16.7% were moderate, and 73.3% were severing level. Cough severity levels were similar to dyspnea levels. After applying the prostrate position and coughing exercises, the levels of dyspnea and coughing improved and become as follows after one hour of implementing the prostrate position and coughing exercises become only 13.3% of patients who had severe dyspnea, and the same percentage remained until after four hours while it increased again after seven hours to reach for 80%. As for the level of dyspnea in the control group, it is noticeable that the severe level of dyspnea remained high in all measurements, and it was as follows: 73.3%, 83.3%, 80%, and 60%.

Regarding the level of cough, it is clear that it was also affected by prostrate position and coughing exercises. 73.3% of patients in the experimental group had a severe level of cough in the period before performing the prostrate position and coughing exercises while after one hour of implementing the prostrate position and coughing exercises become only 13.3% of patients who had severe cough and continued to decline until it reached to 6.7 % after four hours of implementing of the prostrate position and coughing exercises, but increased again to 56.7% after seven hours of the interventional protocol.

Table (4-5) Comparison between the mean of the readings of cardiopulmonary parameters, dyspnea level, and cough level for the experimental group and control group:

Variables	Experimental group					Control group				
	Before	After 1	After 2	After 3	p-value (Sig.)	Before	After 1	After 2	After 3	p-value (Sig.)
SBP (mmHg)	145.4	124.1	132.5	150.1	0.000 (HS)	140.8	138.8	139.1	138.8	0.153 (N.S)
DBP (mmHg)	86	79.1	77	86.1	0.000 (HS)	87.1	87.3	87	85.3	0.153 (N.S)
SpO_2 (%)	82.6	95.1	92.8	82.6	0.000 (HS)	84.4	84.8	85.1	84.	0.398 (N.S)
RR (breath\m minute	35.2	22.8	25	30.16	0.000 (HS)	31.4	30.8	30.4	29.7	0.086 (N.S)
PR (beats/minute)	114.2	83.3	85.7	105.4	0.000 (HS)	103.3	100	100.1	100.6	0.066 (N.S)
Pulse pressure (mm Hg)	56.6	48.4	55.8	59.1	0.021 (S)	53.3	51	50.5	51.5	0.117 (N.S)
MAP (mm Hg)	104.1	94.1	95.9	105.9	0.000 (HS)	107.6	106.4	106.4	105.6	0.071 (N.S)
Cardiac output (Liter/ minute)	16.1	7.2	9.8	12.1	0.041 (S)	15.8	14.7	14.7	15	0.101 (N.S)
Level of Dyspnea	1.9	1.0	1.2	1.8	0.000 (HS)	1.8	1.8	1.8	1.7	0.077 (N.S)
Level of Cough	1.9	1.2	1.2	1.8	0.000 (HS)	1.8	1.8	1.8	1.8	0.166 (N.S)

***Before:** before implementing the intervention; after 1: one hour after implementing the intervention; after 2: four hours after implementing the intervention; after 3: seven hours after implementing the intervention. NS: Non-Significant (P value >0.05); S: Significant (P value ≤0.05- > 0.01) ; HS : Highly Significant (P value ≤0.01).*

This table shows that are a significant statistical differences between the mean of the cardiopulmonary parameters readings, dyspnea level, and cough level for the experimental group, while there is no significant statistical difference between the mean of the readings of cardiopulmonary parameters, dyspnea level, and cough level for the control group.

Table (4-6): Relationship between the effect of prostrate position and patients' cardiopulmonary parameters:

Parameters	Comparative patterns	df	F	p-value	Level
SBP	Sphericity assumed	3	24.889	0.000	HS
	Greenhouse-Geisser	1.861	24.889	0.000	HS
	Huynh-Feldt	1.984	24.889	0.000	HS
	Lower-bound	1.000	24.889	0.000	HS
DBP	Sphericity assumed	3	16.553	0.000	HS
	Greenhouse-Geisser	2.779	16.553	0.000	HS
	Huynh-Feldt	3.000	16.553	0.000	HS
	Lower-bound	1.000	16.553	0.000	HS
SpO_2	Sphericity assumed	3	133.544	0.000	HS
	Greenhouse-Geisser	2.571	133.544	0.000	HS
	Huynh-Feldt	2.843	133.544	0.000	HS
	Lower-bound	1.000	133.544	0.000	HS
RR	Sphericity assumed	3	180.163	0.000	HS
	Greenhouse-Geisser	2.416	180.163	0.000	HS
	Huynh-Feldt	2.651	180.163	0.000	HS
	Lower-bound	1.000	180.163	0.000	HS
PR	Sphericity assumed	3	71.434	0.000	HS
	Greenhouse-Geisser	2.431	71.434	0.000	HS
	Huynh-Feldt	2.669	71.434	0.000	HS
	Lower-bound	1.000	71.434	0.000	HS
PP	Sphericity assumed	3	4.345	0.007	HS
	Greenhouse-Geisser	1.830	4.345	0.021	S
	Huynh-Feldt	1.946	4.345	.0.018	S
	Lower-bound	1.000	4.345	0.046	S
MAP	Sphericity assumed	3	26.304	0.000	HS
	Greenhouse-Geisser	2.137	26.304	0.000	HS
	Huynh-Feldt	2.312	26.304	0.000	HS
	Lower-bound	1.000	26.304	0.000	HS
CO	Sphericity assumed	3	4.453	0.006	HS
	Greenhouse-Geisser	1.066	4.453	0.041	S
	Huynh-Feldt	1.074	4.453	0.040	S
	Lower-bound	1.000	4.453	0.044	S

Level of Dyspnea	Sphericity assumed	3	284.692	0.000	HS
	Greenhouse-Geisser	2.119	284.692	0.000	HS
	Huynh-Feldt	2.291	284.692	0.000	HS
	Lower-bound	1.000	284.692	0.000	HS
Level of Cough	Sphericity assumed	3	147.717	0.000	HS
	Greenhouse-Geisser	2.621	147.717	0.000	HS
	Huynh-Feldt	2.905	147.717	0.000	HS
	Lower-bound	1.000	147.717	0.000	HS

df=Degree of Freedom; F=F-statistics; NS: NS: Non-Significant (P value >0.05); S: Significant (P value ≤0.05- > 0.01) ; HS : Highly Significant (P value ≤0.01).

Repeated Measures ANOVA test was used to determine the difference in the mean of cardiopulmonary parameters scores, level of dyspnea, and severity of cough across four different time periods, and Greenhouse Geisser shows that there is a statistically significant difference in all of these parameters across these four different times at p-value of <0.05.

Table (4-7): Pairwise comparisons of the SBP readings under the effect of prostrate position and coughing exercises between the four measurements periods among the experimental group:

(I) time	(J) time	Mean Difference (I-J)	Std. Error	p-value	Sig.
1	2	21.267*	2.745	0.000	HS
	3	12.933*	4.456	0.007	HS
	4	-.437-	4.275	0.277	NS
2	1	-21.267-*	2.745	0.000	HS
	3	-8.333-*	2.799	0.006	HS
	4	-26.000-*	2.871	0.000	HS
3	1	-12.933-*	4.456	0.007	HS
	2	8.333*	2.799	0.006	HS
	4	-17.667-*	2.557	0.000	HS
4	1	4.733	4.275	0.277	NS
	2	26.000*	2.871	0.000	HS
	3	17.667*	2.557	0.000	HS

Based on estimated marginal means the mean difference is significant at the 0.05 level. NS: Non-Significant (P value >0.05); S: Significant (P value ≤0.05- > 0.01) ; HS : Highly Significant (P value ≤0.01). **(I) time** = The measurement to which it is compared. **(J) time** = Measurements that compare to the main measurement

The pairwise comparisons table shows that there was a highly significant difference in SBP readings between the periods of the application of the interventional protocol (prostrate position and coughing exercises) and one hour after application of the interventional protocol at P-value of 0.000, it represents that the SBP readings before applying the interventional protocol was greater than one hour after applying it, which can be seen from mean difference (I-J) column. There was also a highly significant difference in SBP readings between the period of before applying the interventional protocol and four hours after applying it at P-value of 0.007. Furthermore, it represents that the SBP readings before applying the interventional protocol was greater than four hours after applying it, which can be seen from mean difference (I-J) column. While there was no significant difference in SBP readings between before applying the interventional protocol and seven hours after applying it at p-value of 0.277.

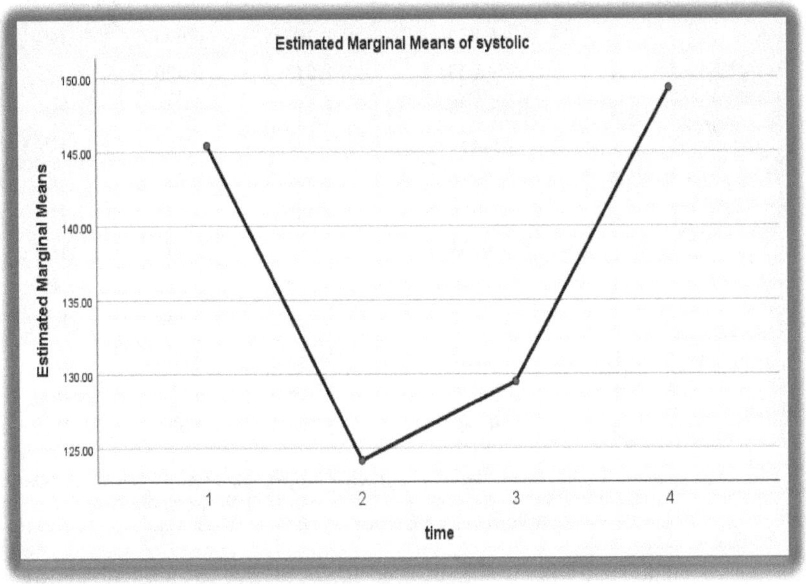

Figure (4-1): Profile plot of SBP readings under the effect of the prostrate position and coughing exercises of the experimental group:

The Profile Plot shows the SBP readings before the application of prostrate position and coughing exercises were greater than the next two readings {one hour and four hours after applying it}. It is also shown, that the effects of prostration position and coughing exercises are disappeared after seven hours of implementing the prostrate position and coughing exercises, as shown in the fourth reading, this indicates that the interventional protocol was effective.

Table (4-8): Pairwise comparisons of the DBP readings under the effect of prostrate position and coughing exercises between the four measurements periods among the experimental group:

(I) time	(J) time	Mean Difference (I-J)	Std. Error	p-value	Sig.
1	2	6.867*	1.703	0.000	HS
	3	9.033*	1.643	0.000	HS
	4	-.133-	1.411	0.925	NS
2	1	-6.867-*	1.703	0.000	HS
	3	2.167	1.809	0.241	NS
	4	-7.000-*	1.459	0.000	HS
3	1	-9.033-*	1.643	0.000	HS
	2	-2.167-	1.809	0.241	NS
	4	-9.167-*	1.763	0.000	HS
4	1	.133	1.411	0.925	NS
	2	7.000*	1.459	0.000	HS
	3	9.167*	1.763	0.000	HS

Based on estimated marginal means the mean difference is significant at the 0.05 level. NS: Non-Significant (P value >0.05); S: Significant (P value ≤0.05- > 0.01) ; HS : Highly Significant (P value ≤0.01). **(I) time** = The measurement to which it is compared. **(J) time** = Measurements that compare to the main measurement

The pairwise comparisons table shows a highly significant difference in DBP readings between the periods of before the application of the interventional protocol (prostrate position and coughing exercises) and one hour after the interventional protocol, and one hour after the application of the interventional protocol at a p-value of 0.000, it represents that the DBP readings before applying the interventional protocol was greater than one hour after applying it, which can be seen from mean difference (I-J) column. There was also a highly significant difference in DBP readings between the period of before applying the interventional protocol, and four hours after the interventional protocol at a p-value of 0.000, it represents that the DBP readings before applying the interventional protocol were greater than four hours after applying it, which can be seen from mean difference (I-J) column. While there was no significant difference in DBP readings between the period of before applying the interventional protocol and seven hours after the interventional protocol at p-value of 0. 92.

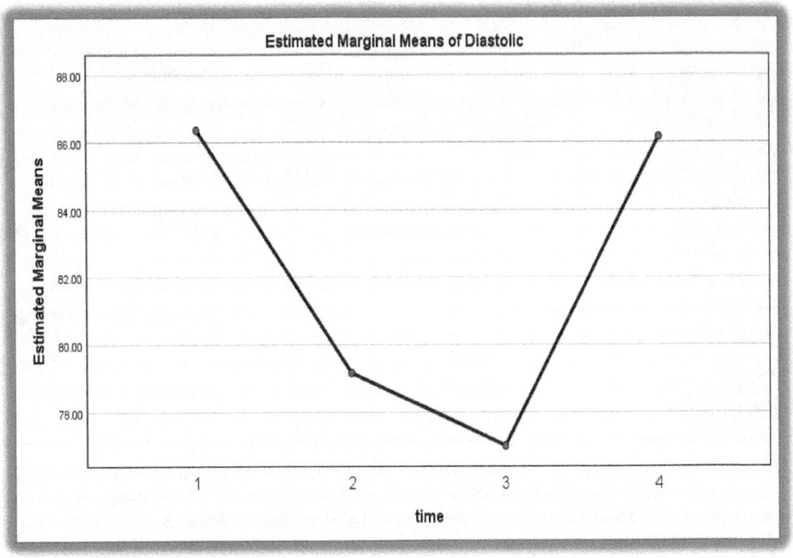

Figure (4-2): Profile plot of DBP readings under the effect of the prostrate position and coughing exercises of the experimental group:

The Profile Plot shows that the DBP readings before applying the interventional protocol (prostrate position and coughing exercises) were greater than the second and third readings. It also shows that the effect of prostrate position and coughing exercises disappeared in the seven hours after applying the prostrate position and coughing exercises, as shown in the fourth reading.

Table (4-9): Pairwise comparisons of the oxygen saturation readings under the effect of prostrate position and coughing exercises between the four measurements periods among the experimental group:

(I) time	(J) time	Mean Difference (I-J)	Std. Error	p-value	Sig.
1	2	-12.500-*	0.845	0.000	HS
	3	-10.167-*	0.807	0.000	HS
	4	-.033-	0.898	0.971	NS
2	1	12.500*	0.845	0.000	HS
	3	2.333*	0.535	0.000	HS
	4	12.467*	0.838	0.000	HS
3	1	10.167*	0.807	0.000	HS
	2	-2.333-*	0.535	0.000	HS
	4	10.133*	0.871	0.000	HS
4	1	.033	0.898	0.971	NS
	2	-12.467-*	0.838	0.000	HS
	3	-10.133-*	0.871	0.000	HS

Based on estimated marginal means the mean difference is significant at the 0.05 level. NS: Non-Significant (P value >0.05); S: Significant (P value ≤0.05- > 0.01) ; HS : Highly Significant (P value ≤0.01). **(I) time** = The measurement to which it is compared. **(J) time** = Measurements that compare to the main measurement

Pairwise comparisons table shows that there was a highly significant difference in oxygen saturation readings between the period of before apply the interventional protocol (prostrate position and coughing exercises) and one hour after applying at P- value of 0.000, it represents that the oxygen saturation readings before applying the interventional protocol was lesser than one hour after applying it, which can be seen from mean difference (I-J) column. There was also a highly significant difference in oxygen saturation readings between the period of before applying the interventional protocol and four hours after applying at P- value of 0.000, it represents that the oxygen saturation readings before applying the interventional protocol was lesser than four hours after applying it, which can be seen from mean difference (I-J) column. While there was no significant difference in oxygen saturation readings between the between the period of before applying the interventional protocol and seven hours after applying the interventional protocol at p- value of 0. 971.

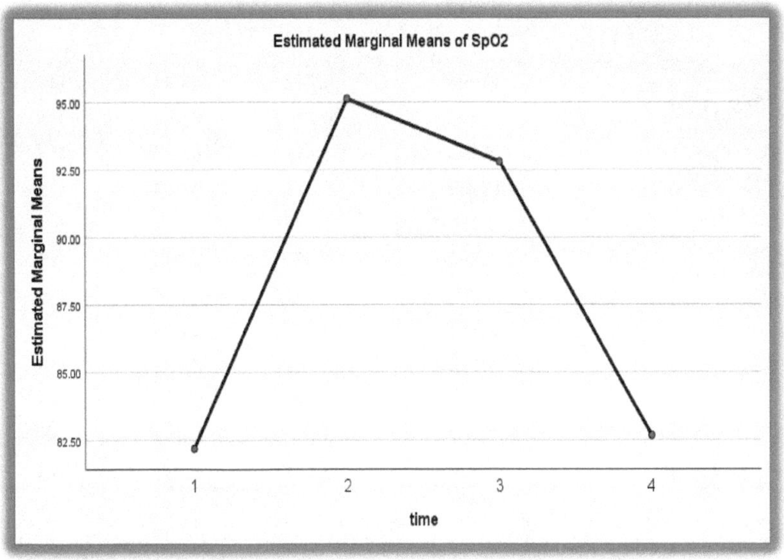

Figure (4-3): Profile plot of oxygen saturation readings under the effect of the prostrate position and coughing exercises of the experimental group:

The Profile Plot shows that the oxygen saturation readings before applying the interventional protocol (prostrate position and coughing exercises) was less than the second and third readings. It is also shows that the effect of the interventional protocol disappears after seven hours of implementing the protocol, as shown in the fourth reading.

Table (4-10): Pairwise comparisons of the RR readings under the effect of prostrate position and coughing exercises between the four measurements periods among the experimental group:

(I) time	(J) time	Mean Difference (I-J)	Std. Error	p-value	Sig.
1	2	12.400*	0.711	0.000	HS
	3	10.133*	0.531	0.000	HS
	4	5.033*	0.490	0.000	HS
2	1	-12.400-*	0.711	0.000	HS
	3	-2.267-*	0.647	0.002	HS
	4	-7.367-*	0.651	0.000	HS
3	1	-10.133-*	0.531	0.000	HS
	2	2.267*	0.647	0.002	HS
	4	-5.100-*	0.411	0.000	HS
4	1	-5.033-*	0.490	0.000	HS
	2	7.367*	0.651	0.000	HS
	3	5.100*	0.411	0.000	HS

Based on estimated marginal means the mean difference is significant at the 0.05 level. NS: Non-Significant (P value >0.05); S: Significant (P value ≤0.05- > 0.01) ; HS : Highly Significant (P value ≤0.01). **(I) time** = The measurement to which it is compared. **(J) time** = Measurements that compare to the main measurement

Pairwise comparisons table shows that there was a highly significant difference in RR readings between the period of before applying the interventional protocol (prostrate position and coughing exercises) and one hour after applying the interventional protocol at P- value of 0.000, it represents that the RR readings before applying interventional protocol was greater than one hour after applying it, which can be seen from mean difference (I-J) column. There was also a highly significant difference in RR readings between the period of before applying the interventional protocol and four hours after applying at P- value of 0.000, it represents that the RR readings before applying the interventional protocol was greater than four hours after applying it, which can be seen from mean difference (I-J) column.

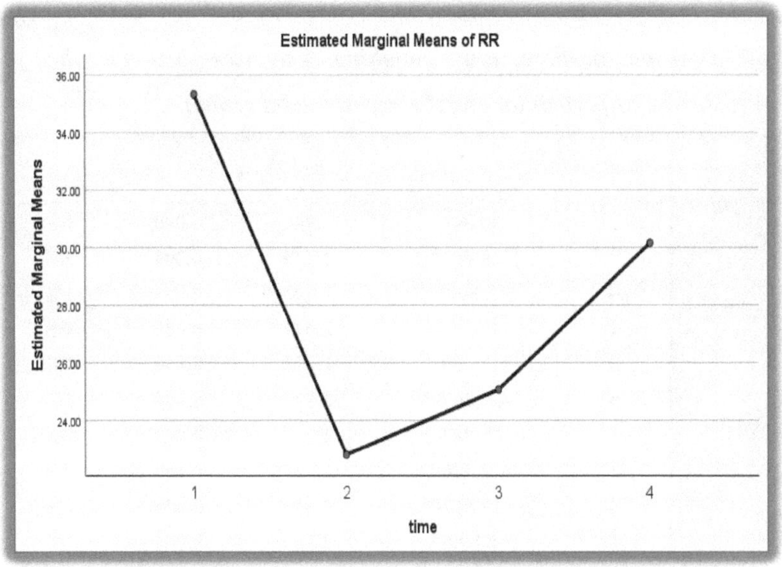

Figure (4-4): Profile plot of RR readings under the effect of the prostrate position and coughing exercises of the experimental group:

The Profile Plot shows that the RR readings before applying the interventional protocol (prostrate position and coughing exercises) were greater than the second and third readings. It also shows that the effect of prostration disappears after seven hours of implementing the interventional protocol, as shown in the fourth reading.

Table (4-11): Pairwise comparisons of the PR readings under the effect of prostrate position and coughing exercises between the four measurements periods among the experimental group:

(I) time	(J) time	Mean Difference (I-J)	Std. Error	p-value	Sig.
1	2	30.867*	2.944	0.000	HS
	3	28.467*	2.750	0.000	HS
	4	8.800*	2.700	0.003	HS
2	1	-30.867-*	2.944	0.000	HS
	3	-2.400-	1.622	0.150	NS
	4	-22.067-*	2.397	0.000	HS
3	1	-28.467-*	2.750	0.000	HS
	2	2.400	1.622	0.150	NS
	4	-19.667-*	2.486	0.000	HS
4	1	-8.800-*	2.700	0.003	HS
	2	22.067*	2.397	0.000	HS
	3	19.667*	2.486	0.000	HS

Based on estimated marginal means the mean difference is significant at the 0.05 level. NS: Non-Significant (P value >0.05); S: Significant (P value ≤0.05- > 0.01) ; HS : Highly Significant (P value ≤0.01). **(I) time** = The measurement to which it is compared. **(J) time** = Measurements that compare to the main measurement

Pairwise comparisons table shows that there was a highly significant difference in PR readings between the period of before applying the interventional protocol (prostrate position and coughing exercises) and one hour after applying at P- value of 0.000, it represents that the PR readings before applying the interventional protocol was greater than one hour after applying it, which can be seen from mean difference (I-J) column. There was also a highly significant difference in PR readings between the period of before applying the interventional protocol and four hours after applying at P- value of 0.000, it represents that the PR readings before applying the interventional protocol was greater than four hours after applying it, which can be seen from mean difference (I-J) column.

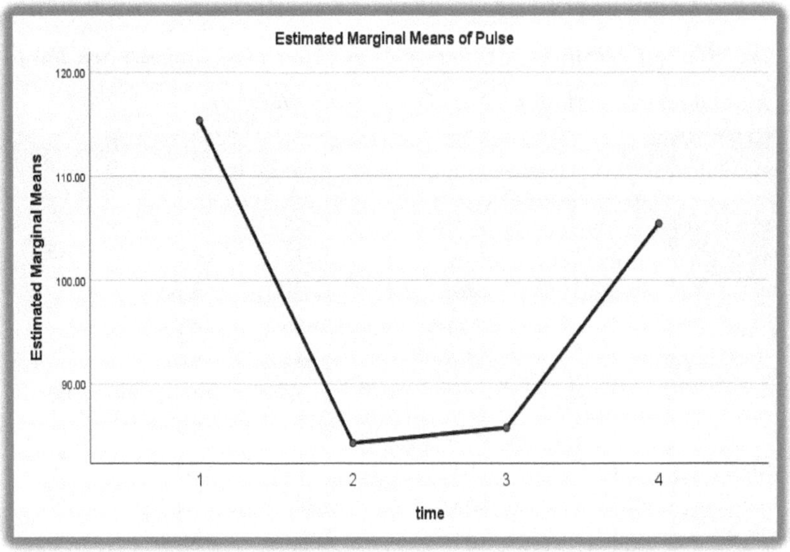

Figure (4-5): Profile plot of PR readings under the effect of the prostrate position and coughing exercises of the experimental group:

This figure shows that the PR reading in the period before applying the interventional protocol (prostrate position and coughing exercises) was greater than the second and third readings. It also shows that the effect of interventional protocol disappears after seven hours of implementing the protocol, as shown in the fourth reading.

Table (4-12): Pairwise comparisons of the pulse pressure readings under the effect of prostrate position and coughing exercises between the four measurements periods among the experimental group:

(I) time	(J) time	Mean Difference (I-J)	Std. Error	p-value	Sig.
1	2	8.200*	2.656	0.004	HS
	3	0.800	4.122	0.847	NS
	4	-2.533-	1.971	0.209	NS
2	1	-8.200-*	2.656	0.004	HS
	3	-7.400-*	2.984	0.019	S
	4	-10.733-*	2.426	0.000	HS
3	1	-.800-	4.122	0.847	NS
	2	7.400*	2.984	0.019	S
	4	-3.333-	4.007	0.412	NS
4	1	2.533	1.971	0.209	NS
	2	10.733*	2.426	0.000	HS
	3	3.333	4.007	0.412	NS

Based on estimated marginal means the mean difference is significant at the 0.05 level. NS: Non-Significant (P value >0.05); S: Significant (P value ≤0.05- > 0.01) ; HS : Highly Significant (P value ≤0.01). **(I) time** = The measurement to which it is compared. **(J) time** = Measurements that compare to the main measurement

The pairwise comparisons table shows that there was a highly significant difference in pulse pressure readings between the period before applying the interventional protocol (prostrate position and coughing exercises) and the second reading (one hour after applying the interventional protocol) at a p-value of 0.004. It was represented that the pulse pressure readings before applying the interventional protocol were greater than the second readings, which can be seen from the mean difference (I-J) column. While there was no significant difference in pulse pressure readings between the period before applying interventional protocol and the third reading (four hours after applying interventional protocol) at a p-value of 0.847 and the fourth reading at a p-value of 0.209.

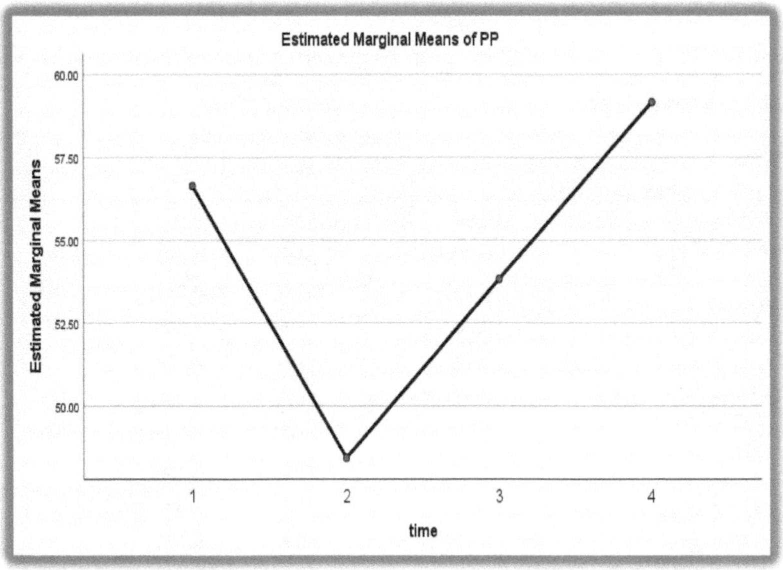

Figure (4-6): Profile plot of pulse pressure readings under the effect of the prostrate position and coughing exercises of the experimental group:

The Profile Plot shows that the pulse pressure readings before applying the interventional protocol (prostrate position and coughing exercises) was greater than the second readings. It is also shows that the effect of prostrate position and coughing exercises disappears after four hours of implementing the protocol, as shown in the third and fourth reading.

Table (4-13): Pairwise comparisons of the MAP readings under the effect of prostrate position and coughing exercises between the four measurements periods among the experimental group:

(I) time	(J) time	Mean Difference (I-J)	Std. Error	p-value	Sig.
1	2	10.067*	1.530	0.000	HS
	3	8.233*	2.230	0.001	HS
	4	-1.767-	1.608	0.281	NS
2	1	-10.067-*	1.530	0.000	HS
	3	-1.833-	1.482	0.226	NS
	4	-11.833-*	1.269	0.000	HS
3	1	-8.233-*	2.230	0.001	HS
	2	1.833	1.482	0.226	NS
	4	-10.000-*	1.448	0.000	HS
4	1	1.767	1.608	0.281	NS
	2	11.833*	1.269	0.000	HS
	3	10.000*	1.448	0.000	HS

Based on estimated marginal means the mean difference is significant at the 0.05 level. NS: Non-Significant (P value >0.05); S: Significant (P value ≤0.05- > 0.01) ; HS : Highly Significant (P value ≤0.01). **(I) time** = The measurement to which it is compared. **(J) time** = Measurements that compare to the main measurement

The pairwise comparisons table shows that there was a highly significant difference in MAP readings between the period of the first reading (before applying interventional protocol) and the second reading (one hour after applying interventional protocol) at a p-value of 0.000 and the third reading (four hours after applying interventional protocol) at a p-value of 0.001, while there was no significant difference in MAP readings between before applying the interventional protocol and forth reading at a p-value of 0.281, it represents that the MAP readings before applying the interventional protocol were greater than second and third readings, which can be seen from mean difference (I-J) column.

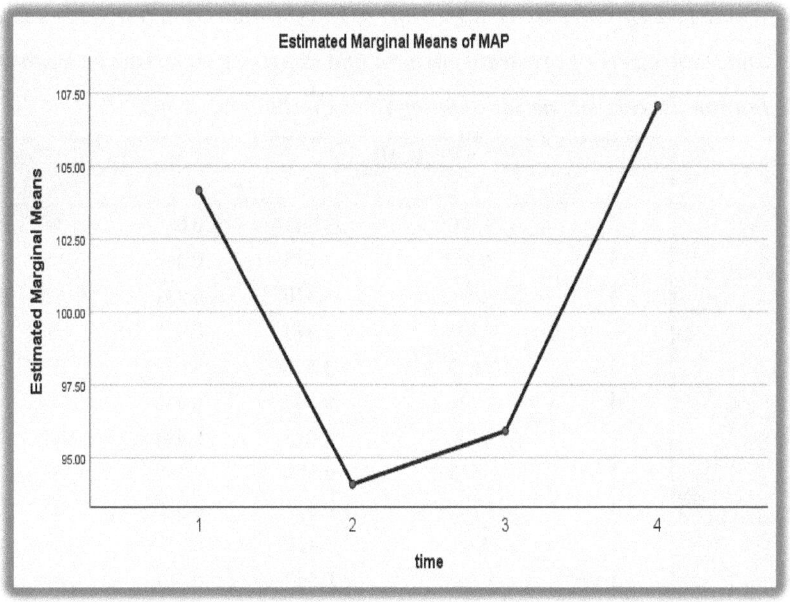

Figure (4-7): Profile plot of MAP readings under the effect of the prostrate position and coughing exercises of the experimental group:

This figure shows that the MAP reading before applying the interventional protocol (prostrate position and coughing exercises) was greater than the second and third readings. It also shows that the effect of prostration disappears after seven hours of implementing the protocol, as shown in the fourth reading.

Table (4-14): Pairwise comparisons of the Cardiac Output (CO) readings under the effect of prostrate position and coughing exercises between the four measurements periods among the experimental group:

(I) time	(J) time	Mean Difference (I-J)	Std. Error	p-value	Sig.
1	2	8.900*	3.544	0.018	S
	3	6.267	3.615	0.094	NS
	4	4.000	3.420	0.252	NS
2	1	-8.900-*	3.544	0.018	S
	3	-2.633-*	0.588	0.000	HS
	4	-4.900-*	0.547	0.000	HS
3	1	-6.267-	3.615	0.094	NS
	2	2.633*	0.588	0.000	HS
	4	-2.267-*	0.573	0.000	HS
4	1	-4.000-	3.420	0.252	NS
	2	4.900*	0.547	0.000	HS
	3	2.267*	0.573	0.000	HS

Based on estimated marginal means the mean difference is significant at the 0.05 level. NS: Non-Significant (P value >0.05); S: Significant (P value ≤0.05- > 0.01) ; HS : Highly Significant (P value ≤0.01). **(I) time** = The measurement to which it is compared. **(J) time** = Measurements that compare to the main measurement

The pairwise comparisons table shows that there was a highly significant difference in CO readings between the period of the first reading (before applying the interventional protocol) and the second reading (one hour after applying the interventional protocol) at a p-value of 0.018. While there was no significant difference in CO readings between the period before applying the interventional protocol and two other readings, at the third reading (four hours after applying the interventional protocol) at a p-value of 0.094, and at the fourth reading at a p-value of 0.252). It represents that the CO readings before applying the interventional protocol were greater than the second readings, which can be seen from Mean Difference (I-J) column.

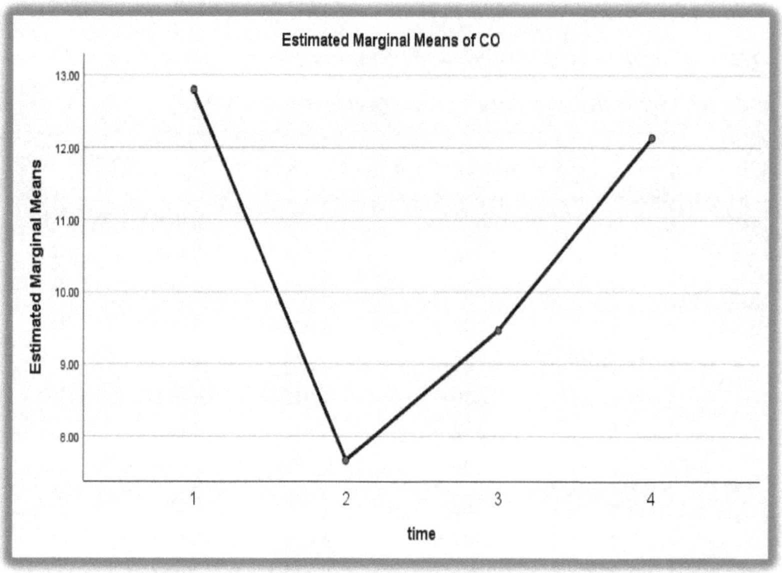

Figure (4-8): Profile plot of CO readings under the effect of the prostrate position and coughing exercises of the experimental group:

This figure shows that the CO readings before applying the interventional protocol (prostrate position and coughing exercises) were greater than the second readings. It also shown that the effect of interventional protocol disappears after four hours, as shown in the third and fourth reading.

Table (4-15): Pairwise comparisons of the level of dyspnea under the effect of prostrate position and coughing exercises between the four measurements periods among the experimental group:

(I) time	(J) time	Mean Difference (I-J)	Std. Error	p-value	Sig.
1	2	.897*	0.028	0.000	HS
	3	.676*	0.034	0.000	HS
	4	.087*	0.029	0.000	HS
2	1	-.897-*	0.028	0.000	HS
	3	-.221-*	0.049	0.000	HS
	4	-.810-*	0.042	0.000	HS
3	1	-.676-*	0.034	0.000	HS
	2	.221*	0.049	0.000	HS
	4	-.589-*	0.035	0.000	HS
4	1	-.087-*	0.029	0.000	HS
	2	.810*	0.042	0.000	HS
	3	.589*	0.035	0.000	HS

Based on estimated marginal means the mean difference is significant at the 0.05 level. NS: Non-Significant (P value >0.05); S: Significant (P value ≤0.05- > 0.01) ; HS : Highly Significant (P value ≤0.01). **(I) time** = The measurement to which it is compared. **(J) time** = Measurements that compare to the main measurement

The pairwise comparisons table shows that there was a highly significant difference in the levels of dyspnea between the first time period (before applying the interventional protocol) and the next second time period (one hour after applying the interventional protocol) at a p-value of 0.000, also with the third time period (four hours after applying interventional protocol) at a p-value of 0.000. It represents that the dyspnea level score before applying the interventional protocol (prostrate position and coughing exercises) was greater than the next second time, which can be seen from the mean difference (I-J) column.

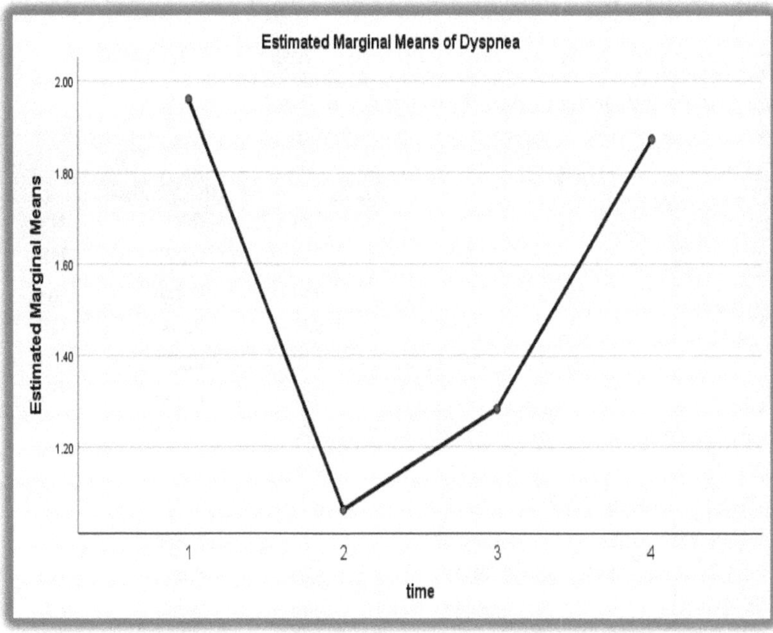

Figure (4-9): Profile plot of level of dyspnea under the effect of the prostrate position and coughing exercises of the experimental group:

The Profile Plot shows that the level of dyspnea before applying the interventional protocol (prostrate position and coughing exercises) was greater than the next second times. It is also shows that the effect of the interventional protocol does not disappears after four hours of implementing the protocol, as shown in the third time.

Table (4-16): Pairwise comparisons of the cough severity under the effect of prostrate position and coughing exercises between the four measurements periods among the experimental group:

(I) time	(J) time	Mean Difference (I-J)	Std. Error	p-value	Sig.
1	2	.700*	.037	0.000	HS
	3	.653*	.046	0.000	HS
	4	.093*	.042	0.036	S
2	1	-.700-*	.037	0.000	HS
	3	-.047-	.040	0.257	NS
	4	-.607-*	.049	0.000	HS
3	1	-.653-*	.046	0.000	HS
	2	.047	.040	0.257	NS
	4	-.560-*	.040	0.000	HS
4	1	-.093-*	.042	0.036	S
	2	.607*	.049	0.000	HS
	3	.560*	.040	0.000	HS

***Based on estimated marginal means the mean difference is significant at the 0.05 level. NS: Non-Significant (P value >0.05); S: Significant (P value ≤0.05- > 0.01) ; HS : Highly Significant (P value ≤0.01).*(I) time** = The measurement to which it is compared. **(J) time** = Measurements that compare to the main measurement

The pairwise comparisons table shows that there was a highly significant difference in the severity of cough scores between the first time period (before applying the interventional protocol) and the next second time at a p-value of 0.000, and with the second time period (one hour after applying interventional protocol) at a p-value of 0.000, and with the period of the third time (four hours after applying interventional protocol). It represents that the cough severity level score before applying the interventional protocol (prostrate position and coughing exercises) was greater than the next second time, which can be seen from the mean difference (I-J) column.

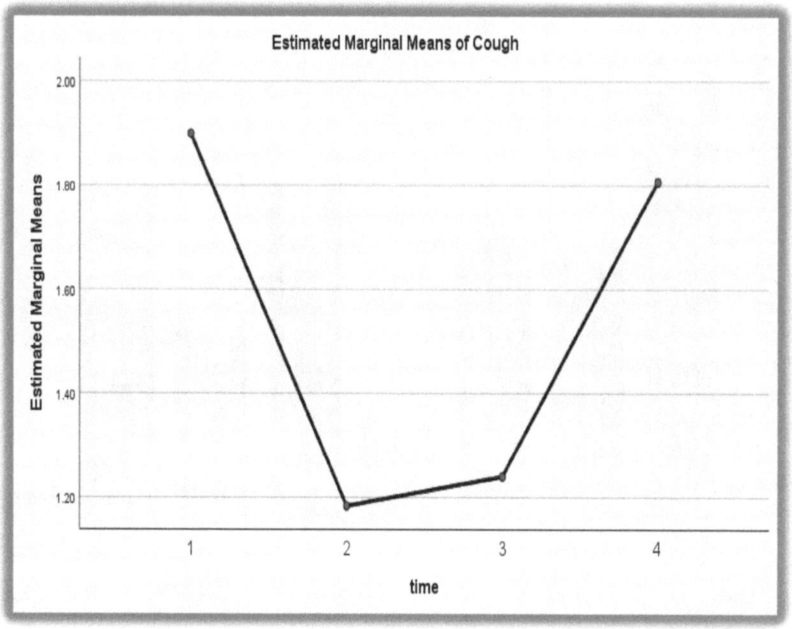

Figure (4-10): Profile plot of severity of cough under the effect of the prostrate position and coughing exercises of the experimental group:

The Profile Plot shows that the cough severity level scores in the period of before applying the interventional protocol (prostrate position and coughing exercises) was greater than the next second scores. It also shows that the effect of prostrate position not disappears after four hours of implementing the protocol, as shown in the third time.

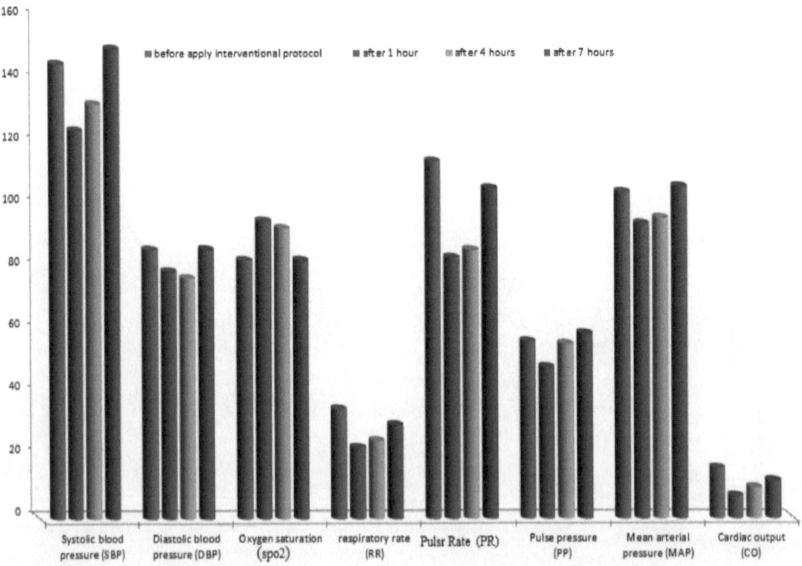

Figure (4-11): Effect of prostrate position and coughing exercises upon cardiopulmonary parameters among the experimental group:

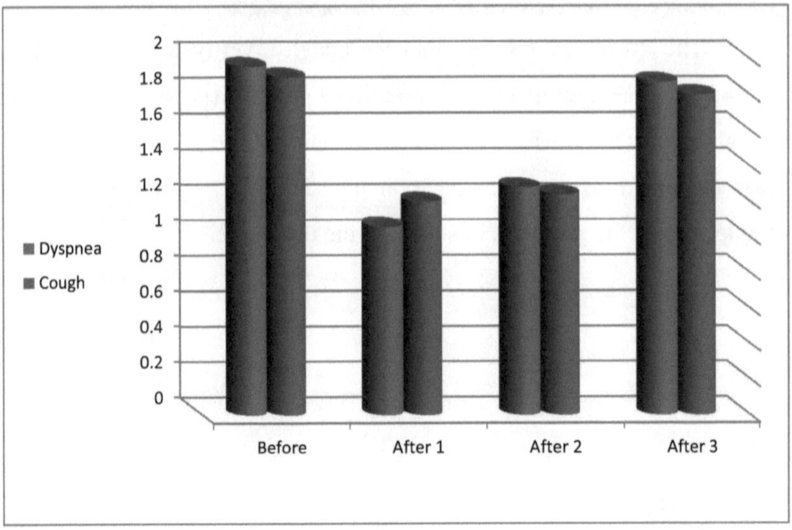

Figure (4-12): Effect of prostrate position and coughing exercises upon level of dyspnea and cough among the experimental group:

Table (4-17): Association between the effect of prostrate position and coughing exercises upon the level of dyspnea, cough severity, and cardiopulmonary parameters among non-intubated COVID-19 patients with their socio-demographic characteristics:

Variables	Age		Gender		Smoking condition		Second-hand smoke		BMI	
	P-value	Sig.	P-value	Sig.	P-value	Sig.	P-value	Sig.	P-value	Sig.
SBP	0.001	HS	0.078	NS	0.039	S	0.065	NS	0.001	HS
DBP	0.009	HS	0.043	S	0.132	NS	0.018	HS	0.002	HS
SpO_2	0.410	NS	0.451	NS	0.015	HS	0.206	NS	0.152	NS
RR	0.005	HS	0.020	S	0.204	NS	0.541	NS	0.013	S
PR	0.013	S	0.052	NS	0.033	S	0.108	NS	0.002	HS
Pulse pressure	0.089	NS	0.078	NS	0.098	NS	0.112	NS	0.227	NS
MAP	0.061	NS	0.135	NS	0.074	NS	0.250	NS	0.007	HS
CO	0.163	NS	0.144	NS	0.007	HS	0.012	S	0.000	HS
Level of Dyspnea	0.138	NS	0.333	NS	0.497	NS	0.043	S	0.011	S
Cough Severity	0.001	HS	0.088	NS	0.277	NS	0.071	NS	0.528	NS

NS: Non-Significant (P value >0.05); S: Significant (P value ≤0.05- > 0.01) ; HS : Highly Significant (P value ≤0.01).

Chi-square test table shows there was a statistically significant association between the improvement in the SBP with age group, smoking condition, and BMI. Also, there was a statistically significant association between the improvement in the DBP with age group, gender, second-hand smoke, and BMI. In addition to that, the improvement in SpO_2 reading had a statistically significant association with the smoking conditions. There was an association between the improvement effect in the RR with age group, gender, and BMI. And there was an association between the improvement in the PR with age group, smoking condition, and BMI. Furthermore, the improvement in the MAP had an association with BMI. Also, there was an association between the improvement in the CO with smoking conditions, second-hand smoke, and BMI. The improvement in the level of dyspnea has been shown to be associated with second-hand smoke, and BMI. Finally, this table shows that there was found a statistically significant association between the cough severity with the patients age group.

Table (4-18): Association between the effect of prostrate position and coughing exercises upon the level of dyspnea, cough severity, and cardiopulmonary parameters among COVID-19 patients with their clinical data:

Variables	Chronic diseases		Current medication history						Infected part of the lung		Percentage of the affected area		The period since the first appearance of symptoms		Hospitalization period		Method of oxygenation therapy		Take vaccine condition	
			Using antitussive medications		Using bronchodilat or medications		Using antipyretic medications													
	P-Value	Sig.	P-Value	Sig.	P-Value	Sig.	P-Value	Sig.	P-Value	Sig.	P-Value	Sig.	P-Value	Sig.	P-Value	Sig.	P-Value	Sig.	P-Value	Sig.
SBP	0.036	S	0.154	NS	0.032	S	0.209	NS	0.060	NS	0.025	S	0.031	S	0.011	S	0.397	NS	0.008	HS
DBP	0.010	HS	0.018	HS	0.088	NS	0.254	NS	0.002	HS	0.008	HS	0.002	HS	0.008	HS	0.067	NS	0.018	S
SpO_2	0.020	S	0.769	NS	0.536	NS	0.977	NS	0.016	S	0.051	NS	0.055	NS	0.155	NS	0.387	NS	0.811	NS
RR	0.001	HS	0.209	NS	0.016	S	0.769	NS	0.000	HS	0.034	S	0.028	S	0.004	HS	0.049	S	0.945	NS
PR	0.008	HS	0.052	NS	0.091	NS	0.286	NS	0.003	HS	0.013	S	0.028	S	0.035	S	0.052	NS	0.052	NS
Pulse pressure	0.001	HS	0.008	HS	0.023	S	0.455	NS	0.011	S	0.231	NS	0.009	HS	0.050	S	0.049	S	0.945	NS
MAP	0.126	NS	0.915	NS	0.091	NS	0.052	NS	0.017	S	0.041	S	0.087	NS	0.106	NS	0.052	NS	0.052	NS
CO	0.003	HS	0.109	NS	0.132	NS	0.012	HS	0.003	HS	0.017	S	0.007	HS	0.001	HS	0.087	NS	0.012	S
Level of Dyspnea	0.148	NS	0.925	NS	0.077	NS	0.209	NS	0.041	S	0.201	NS	0.045	S	0.274	NS	0.193	NS	0.018	S
Cough Severity	0.056	NS	0.245	NS	0.245	NS	0.425	NS	0.025	S	0.081	S	0.073	NS	0.062	NS	0.232	NS	0.970	NS

NS: Non-Significant (P value >0.05); S: Significant (P value ≤0.05- > 0.01) ; HS : Highly Significant (P value ≤0.01)

Chi-square test table shows that there was a significant association between the improvement in the SBP and chronic disease, the using of bronchodilators medications, the percentage of the affected area, the period since the first appearance of symptoms, hospitalization period, and COVID-19 vaccination. The improvement in the DPB had statistical significant with chronic disease, the using of antitussive medications, infected part of the lung, percentage of the affected area, the period since the first appearance of symptoms, hospitalization period, and take COVID-19 vaccination. There was an association between the improvement in the SpO_2 and chronic disease, the infected part of the lung, the percentage of the affected area, and the period since the first appearance of symptoms. There was an association between the improvement in the RR and chronic disease, the using of bronchodilators medications, infected part of the lung, percentage of the affected area, the period since the first appearance of symptoms, hospitalization period, and method of oxygenation therapy. In addition to that, there was an association between the improvements in the PR with chronic disease, the using of antitussive medications, infected part of the lung, percentage of the affected area, the period since the first appearance of symptoms, hospitalization period, method of oxygenation therapy, and COVID-19 vaccination. The improvement in the level of dyspnea have been shows to be associated with the infected part of the lung, the period since the first appearance of symptoms, and COVID-19 vaccination status. As for the association between the improvement in the cough severity and some clinical data, this table exposed that there was a significant association with the infected part of the lung and percentage of the affected area.

Chapter five

Discussion

Chapter five
Discussion of the results

It is possible to control the severity of the infection with COVID-19 and reduce its complications and decrease the mortality rate through improving oxygenation and ensuring high gas exchange, as well as reducing the severity of cough associated with COVID-19. A 60 male and female patients who were confirmed to have COVID-19 participated in this study to investigate the effect of prostrate position and coughing exercises upon the level of dyspnea, persistent cough, and cardiopulmonary parameters among non-intubated patients with COVID-19.

5.1. Discussion of socio-demographical characteristics of COVID-19 patients:

Concerning the socio-demographic characteristics of participants as shown in table (4-1), the results reveals that the most participants were located in the age group of $\geq$ 60 years it represent of 63.3% for experimental group and 66.6% for control group. Boehmer, et al., (2020) conducted a retrospective study in USA on hospitalized patients infected with COVID- 19 who reported that the incidence of COVID-19 was highest in patients aged 20 to 29 years and accounted for about more than 20%. The researcher believes that the number of elderly COVID-19 patients in his sample had increased due to the weak immunity of those people. Mueller, et al., (2020) described that "the aging innate immune system" that led to their intolerance to the complications of the disease, which led to their hospitalization, unlike the young people group who have good immunity and a healthy body that helps them withstand the disease.

As for gender, the results of the study indicated that 60 % of participants were males, and 40% were females for experimental group, while in control group was 46.7 % were males and 53.3 % were females. The researcher show that this convergence in the percentages of sample by gender (males and females) means that there were no clear differences between the genders and that the virus infects both gender with similar chances. The results of this study agree with a study conducted by Jin, et al., (2020) stated that the prevalence of COVID-19 among women and men was similar, they were emphasized that the men patients with COVID-19 were at high risk for worse outcomes, independent of aging. Conversely, a study done by Marik, et al., (2021) exposed that the COVID-19 is severe in males regardless of age or other diseases although there are several studies indicating that males had the highest inflammatory response. This is attributed to the inhibition of the production of pro-inflammatory cytokines by Estrogens which is the main mechanism to explain the gender differential among COVID-19 patients. A study conducted by Garcia, et al., (2021) stated that the ratio of men infected by COVID-19 was 50.4% and women were 49.6% this means that there was a similarity in the incidence rate between the genders.

With regard to smoking status, the study indicated that 76.7% of experimental group and 66.7% of control group were non-smokers, which means that the spread of the disease is not limited to smokers person only, but includes all groups, this finding agrees with the results of the study that conducted by Vardavas and Nikitara, (2020) stated that 27.3% of patients with a smoking history. Patanavanich and Glantz, (2021) reported that smoking cessation should be a priority for the prevention of COVID-19 infection because smoking is one of the most important risk factors of COVID-19 infection. The effect of smoking was evident in young patients. The researcher attribute the reason for the low rates of smoking in the sample to the presence of nearly half of the sample from women, and in the eastern society the smoking rate for women is very limited.

Concerning the exposure to second-hand smoke, the study results reveal that 80 % of experimental group and 76.7% of control group were exposure to second-hand smoke. This ratio was because that exposure to second-hand smoke exposure was harmful especially to children, young people, and elderly. They inhale double the amount of dust compared with adults, thus inhaling more smoke containing dust particles. This increases the rate of harm to the lungs, making it more vulnerable to the invasion of microorganisms, especially the Corona virus (Osinibi, et al., 2021). The mortality rate in males was 4.7% while in women was 2.6% these differences could be due to the differences in patterns of smoking and prevalence between males and females (Garcia, et al., 2021).

5.2. Discussion of BMI among COVID-19 patients:

BMI has strong link with severity of COVID-19 as shown in the table (4-2) the result indicates that 53.3% of patients for the experimental group and 46.7% for the control group were suffering from obesity class I who were located in the group at BMI of 30-34.9, these results agree with the study which done by Raisi-Estabragh, et al., (2020) exposed that the highest BMI was accompanied by a COVID-19 infection among patients who have moderate to severe symptoms. The researcher show that he reasons for the weight gain of patients who enrolled in the study were attributed to two things: the first reason, that nearly half of the sample was women. The weight gain among elderly Iraqi women was very high (Al Tawil, et al., 2007). The second reason that the accumulation of adipose tissues causes mechanical changes in organs and tissues that cause severe impairment of somebody's systems which results in severe complications (Hendren, et al., 2021).

5.3. Discussion of clinical data of COVID-19 Patients: Clinical data has strong link with severity of COVID-19, according to the study's findings as illustrated in table (4-3), it is show that 36.7% of the patients in experimental and control groups do not have any chronic diseases. Due to the convergence of some percentages, this percent does not represent an absolute majority; especially since approximately one-third of the patients suffer from asthma. Exacerbations of asthma were more likely to be caused by other triggers, such as allergens or virus exposure, or even stopping taking prescription drugs on a regular basis. The exacerbation of asthma increases with the increase in the number of triggers, and because the Coronavirus is one of the causes of an asthma attack and other respiratory problems, it increases the complications of asthma. As a result, asthmatic patients infected with the Coronavirus experience significant consequences, increasing their odds of being hospitalized and lengthening their stay (The researcher). According to Adir, et al., (2021), chronic or continued use of systemic corticosteroids for asthma therapy before COVID-19 infection is the greatest risk factor for low outcomes and reduced survival in asthma patients. Another study by Lee, et al., (2020) found that asthma is not considered a risk factor for a bad COVID-19 infection outcome. However, asthmatic patients who had an acute episode in the year before to COVID-19 had a higher COVID-19related death rate, especially in the elderly and male gender.

As for the medications used to treat COVID-19 complications, it is obvious that the absolute majority of patients use cough suppressants, antipyretics, and steroid therapy. While we find that nearly two-thirds of the sample does not use bronchodilators drugs and this is consistent with what was previously mentioned that only one-third of the sample have asthma. This means that two-thirds of the sample did not suffer from severe bronchoconstriction.

Regarding the affected part of the lung, we found that 43.3% of COVID-19 patients in experimental group suffer from hurt in bi lateral - peripheral and central area of lung, and 40% for control group, this results come along with a study conducted by Soldati, et al., (2020) found that after analyzing the available computed tomographic scan (CT-scan) data from COVID-19 patients, there are mostly some confluent and patchy bilateral lesions that resemble ground glass or have a mixed ground glass and consolidative pattern. The lower right lobe of the lung, followed by the lower and upper left lobes, is the most usually afflicted. Castelao, et al., (2021) stated that the ultrasound involvement in COVID-19 infection is heterogeneous and bilateral. The inferior and posterior areas were the most affected lungs parts. the researcher believe that the reason why the majority of patients enrolled in this study suffer from injury was in the Bilateral - peripheral and central areas of the lung it was attributed to what was previously mentioned that the majority of patients were elderly, obese, have asthma, and exposed to second hand smoke, all of these reasons lead to low immunity and the spread of the Coronavirus inside the lung.

Among patients participated in this study, and regarding the percentage of the affected area of the lungs, the results of this study reveals that four-fifths of the experimental group had more than 45% of their lungs are affected, and this was not much different from the control group, where the percentage indicated that half of them suffer from the same percentage damage. This was evident in the study sample because the study was conducted on patients hospitalized and most of those who need to be hospitalized were those who have a very high rate of lung damage (the researcher).

This study showed that 73.3% of the experimental group, and 53.4% of the control group had symptoms for more than seven days before their admission to the hospital for treatment. This indicates the lack of awareness of the majority of society about the seriousness of the complications of COVID-19, (the researcher). The hospitalization period for nearly half of the sample for both experimental and control groups was between 4-6 days. These results come along with the study done by Altuntas, et al., (2021) reported that the average symptom duration was 8 days and the total hospitalization period was 13 days.

Furthermore, a face mask was used by approximately two-thirds of the patients in both the experimental and control groups to administer oxygen. This was attributed to the fact that the patients chosen for the research were non-intubated and not from critical cases, therefore this method of oxygen delivery was suitable for the majority of them. These findings agree with the study conducted by Sartini, et al., (2020) reported that all 62 patients with mild to moderate ARDS were using facemask as noninvasive ventilation to oxygen administration. Furthermore, when it comes to COVID-19 immunization, the results show that 90 % of the experimental group and 96.7 % of the control group do not take the COVID-19 vaccine. This result agrees with the findings of a study conducted by Abdulah (2021) in Dohuk City, Iraq, on 926 COVID-19 patients, which revealed that 83.5% of the patients had not received any type of COVID-19 immunization.

5.4. Discussion of dyspnea and cough levels among the experimental and control group:

Dyspnea and cough are the most common clinical features of COVID-19 as shown in table (4-4) the result in the four measures, indicate that the difference in the levels of dyspnea and cough in experimental and control groups is shown in the first measurement (before performing the prostration position and coughing exercises), it represent that 73.3% of the experimental group have sever dyspnea but after one hour implementing the prostrate position and coughing exercises in an hour, the percentage of severe dyspnea was only 13.3 %, and the same percentage remained until four hours later and then increased to 80 % after seven hours. Regarding to the level of dyspnea in the control group, it is noticeable that the severe level of dyspnea remained high in all four measures, and it was as follows: 73.3%, 83.3%, 80%, and 60% among four periods respectively (before implemented the protocol, one hour after implementing protocol, after four hours, and after seven hours). With regards to the cough severity, it's clear that prostration and coughing exercises had an effect on the cough severity. The experimental group's level of severe cough was 73.3 % in the first measurement (before performing the prostration and coughing exercises), 13.3 % after one hour, and 6.7 % after four hours, but increased to 56.7 % after seven hours. While the proportion of severe coughing in the control group did not change significantly during the four measures 66.7 %, 90 %, 83.3 %, and 80 % respectively. We believe that the decreasing in the level of severe dyspnea in the experimental group is due to lung reversal and allowing the dorsal alveoli to open and participate in the gas exchange process that takes place inside them, in addition to the positive effect of coughing exercises that help the patient get rid of secretions within the bronchial trees that impede the process of breathing and gas exchange. McNicholas et al., (2020), reported that reduced airway closure in dorsal lung areas due to a more uniform gravitational pleural pressure gradient, improved sputum clearance, increases in functional residual capacity, changes in region of diaphragm movement, and blood flow redistribution. Henderson, (2014) conducted a study to investigate the effect of prone position on improving oxygenation and decrease mortality among patients with ARDS stated that ventilation is enhanced in prone position due to changes in pleural pressure and a reduction in the amount of alveoli collapse, and the alveolus will remain open when the intra-alveolar pressure increases. In their study "Awake prone positioning for hypoxemic respiratory failure: past, COVID-19, and prospective," Touchon et al., (2021) found that the prone position reallocates lung densities from the dorsal to the ventral regions. This study found that while COVID-19 may enhance oxygenation in conscious patients in the prone position. Jarosz, et al., (2020) reported that postural drainage is a method of therapy for people who have difficulties expelling large amounts of bronchial secretions. Effective coughing exercises should be done in situations that help with expectoration, cough alleviation, and lung ventilation.

5.5. Discussion of the comparison between the mean of the readings of cardiopulmonary parameters, dyspnea and cough levels:

As shown in table (4-5) the use of prostrate position and coughing exercises among COVID-19 patients revealed that, it is highly advantageous to use prostrate position and coughing exercises to promote breathing patterns and reduce cough severity. The findings show that there is a statistically significant difference between the mean score of SBP, DBP, SpO_2, RR, PR, PP, MAP, CO, dyspnea level and the severity of cough in the experimental group, but there is no statistically significant difference in the control group. The level of dyspnea and the severity of cough in the experimental group were lowered immediately and four hours after applying for the prostrate position and coughing exercises. This was because the location shifted lung densities from dorsal to ventral areas. These findings led directly to the "sponge lung model," in which COVID-19 is characterized by a heavy edematous lung that resembles a wet sponge, causing dyspnea and coughing. Touchon, et al., (2021) found that the prone position reallocates lung densities from the dorsal to the ventral regions. This study revealed that while COVID-19 may increase oxygenation in conscious patients in the prone position, the effect on clinical outcomes and persistence after re-supination have yet to be determined.

The researcher believe that the reversal of the lung in a prostrate position, which is one of the modes of secretion drainage, as well as coughing exercises, helped to remove sputum and sticky mucous secretions from inside the alveoli into the respiratory tracts, making the process of oxygenation easier. The expansion of the lungs, the opening of the alveoli, and the enhancement of gas exchange are all good outcomes of this process. The patient relaxes psychologically as SpO_2 increases and RR decreases, stress relief, and effort during breathing decreases, resulting in lower PR, BP, CO, and other cardiac indicators. The improvement in arterial oxygenation after changing position (implementing prone position) is attributed to increased regional ventilation in dependent lung areas near the diaphragm and reduced pleural pressure (McNicholas, et al., 2020). Because it is one of the movements unique to Muslim prayer, prostration provides psychological comfort to patients. It is the daily method they use for spiritual contact with the Lord, who provides them with reassurance, calmness, and safety, which agrees with a study conducted in Iraq by Ibraheem, et al., (2021), who found that during prostration (Sajdah), psychological satisfaction occurs as a result of their closeness to God, and this has a positive impact on health status. In non-invasive ventilation patients, Sartini, et al. (2020) found a clear statistical difference between SpO_2, PaO_2, and RR before, during, and after the implementation of prone position. According to a study conducted by Mahrous, and Aboelmagd, (2022), the knee-chest position resulted in a significant decrease in RR, PR, and SpO_2. Rossi, et al., (2022) stated that 65% of COVID-19 patients with pneumonia had increased PaO_2/ FiO_2 after implementing of prone position.

5.6. Discussion of the association between the effect of prostrate position and coughing exercises on the cardiopulmonary parameters, level of dyspnea, and cough severity among COVID-19 patients with their socio-demographic characteristics:

The results in table (4-17) show a highly significant association between the effect of prostrate position and coughing exercises and the respondents' socio-demographic characteristics as following: the results of this study exposed that there was association between SBP with age group, smoking condition, and BMI. Also there was a statistically significant association between the improvement in the DBP with age group, gender, second hand smoke, and BMI. The prostrate position has been clearly improved in the SpO_2 reading among smoker patients.

The improvement in the RR after the application of prostrate position has been clearly associated with age, gender, and BMI. And there was an association between the improvement in the HR with age group, smoking condition, and BMI. MAP had improvement association with BMI. There was an association between the effect of prostrate position on CO and smoking condition, second hand smoke, and BMI. There was a statistically significant association between the improvement in the level of dyspnea and secondhand smoke, and BMI. As for the association between cough severity and some socio-demographic data the results in the table (4-17) shows that there was a statistically significant association between the improvement in the cough severity and age group. Sun, et al., (2020) reported that the severity of COVID-19 increased as the aging process progressed. Lee, et al., (2021) found that a link between SOB, secondhand smoking, and BMI. They also stated that gender has an impact on dyspnea. Kwok, et al., (2020) reported that the obese patients had a higher risk for hospitalization with COVID-19 and there was a relationship between increasing values of BMI and the proportion of patients with severe COVID-19.

5.7. Discussion of the association between the effect of prostrate position and coughing exercises on the cardiopulmonary parameters, level of dyspnea, and cough severity among COVID-19 patients with their clinical data:

The result in a table (4-18) reveals a highly significant association between the effects of prostrate position and coughing exercises with the clinical data of the patients. There was association between the improvement in the SBP and chronic disease, bronchodilators, percentage of the affected area, the period since the first appearance of symptoms, hospitalization period, and take vaccine condition. DBP improvement had significant association with chronic disease, antitussive, infected part of the lung, percentage of the affected area, and the period since the first appearance of symptoms, hospitalization period, and take vaccine condition. There was association between the improvement in the SpO_2 with chronic disease, infected part of the lung, percentage of the affected area, and the period since the first appearance of symptoms. There was an association between the improvement in the RR with chronic disease, bronchodilators, infected part of the lung, percentage of the affected area, the period since the first appearance of symptoms, hospitalization period, and method of oxygenation therapy. There was an association between the improvement in the PR with chronic disease, antitussive, infected part of the lung, percentage of the affected area, the period since the first appearance of symptoms, hospitalization period, method of oxygenation therapy, and take vaccine condition. There was significant association between the improvements in the level of dyspnea with infected part of the lung, the period since the first appearance of symptoms, and COVID-19 vaccination status. As for the association between the improvements in the cough severity with some clinical data, this table exposed that there was a significant association between the improvement in the cough and infected part of the lung and percentage of the affected area. Altuntas, et al., (2021) found that there was a significant link between COVID-19 infection with age and chronic disease. And stated that the majority of participants were elderly, and they had hypertension, cardiovascular disease, COPD, and diabetes.

Baysal, et al., (2018), found that the More than two-thirds of patients were elderly, 86% had used a bronchodilator medication, and 93% had used cortisone therapy. In the prone position, there was a significant association between the severity of dyspnea and PR at the p-value of 0.027, while there was no significant association with other hemodynamic parameters (SBP, DBP, RR, and SpO_2). Tripod position affected the severity of dyspnea at the p-value of 0.003 but the SBP, DBP, PR, RR, and SpO_2 were not affected. Khedar, et al., (2021) reported that there was an association between the severity of disease in the first wave and second wave by the presence of differences in requiring supplementary oxygen, using of steroids medications, hospitalization period, and mortality rate.

Chapter Six

Conclusions & Recommendations

Chapter Six

Conclusions and Recommendations

6.1. Conclusion:

The results of this study conclude that:

1. Most of patients with COVID-19 enrolled in this study were elderly, and about half of them were males and the other were females. Non-smokers, but exposed to secondhand smoke.
2. Most of the patients with COVID-19 had a bilateral-peripheral and central lung parts damaged, with a damage rate of more than 45%, and most of them not vaccinated.
3. The absolute majority of inpatients with COVID-19 which enrolled in this study were had sever in level of cough and dyspnea.
4. The prostrate position and coughing exercises are very useful in decreasing the level of dyspnea, the severity of coughing, and improving the cardiopulmonary parameters among non-intubated patients with COVID-19.
5. The positive effect of the prostrate position and coughing exercises lasted for approximately four hours after the application of the interventional protocol.
6. There is a highly significant association between the improvement in the SBP, and DBP reading with the participants' age group, BMI, chronic disease, percentage of the affected area, duration of symptoms, hospitalization period, and COVID-19 vaccination.
7. A highly significant association was found between the improvement effect in the RR, and PR reading with the participants' age, BMI, chronic disease, the use of bronchodilators medications, the infected

part of the lung, percentage of the affected area, duration of symptoms, hospitalization period, and method of O_2 therapy.

8. A highly significant association between the improvement in the CO with the participants' smoking conditions, second-hand smoke, and BMI. And between the improvement in SpO_2 reading with the participants' smoking conditions, chronic disease, the infected part of the lung, the percentage of the affected area, and the duration of symptoms.
9. The improvement in the level of dyspnea has been shown to be associated with the participants' second-hand smoke, BMI, the infected part of the lung, the period since the first appearance of symptoms, and COVID-19 vaccination. And between the improvements in the cough severity with the participants' age group, the infected part of the lung, and the percentage of the affected area.

6.2. Recommendations:

Based on the results and conclusions the researcher suggests the following recommendations:

1. All patients infected with COVID-19 that are suffering from dyspnea and cough should be instructed to perform the prostrate position and coughing exercises for a full one hour every four hours.
2. Patients with COVID-19 should be instructed to perform the prostrate position and coughing exercises to improve their cardiopulmonary parameters.
3. Further studies should be done to confirm the effect of prostrate position on patients with other respiratory diseases.
4. Another study should be conduct to investigate the benefit of the prostrate position and coughing exercises on other cardiopulmonary parameters that were not included in this study such as PaO_2, $PaCO_2$, PH, HCO_3, and FIO_2.

References

References:

1. Abd El Aziz, M., Ibrahim, H., and Elgzar, W. (2016). Effect of Application of Health Belief Model on Pregnant Women' Knowledge and Health Beliefs Regarding Urogenital Infections. *Journal of Nursing and Health Science*. 5 (5): 34-44. DOI: 10.9790/1959-0505013444.
2. Abdulah, D. (2021). Prevalence and correlates of COVID-19 vaccine hesitancy in the general public in Iraqi Kurdistan: A cross sectional study. *Journal of Medical Virology*. *93*: 6722-6731. https://doi.org/10.1002/jmv.27255ABDULAH|6731
3. Adir, Y., Saliba, W., Beurnier, A., and Humbert, M. (2021). Asthma and COVID-19: an update. Eur Respir Rev; 30: 210152. https://doi.org/10.1183/16000617.0152-2021
4. Aeen, F. B., Pakzad, R., Rad, M. G., Abdi, F., Zaheri, F., & Mirzadeh, N. (2021). Effect of prone position on respiratory parameters, intubation and death rate in COVID-19 patients: systematic review and meta-analysis. *Scientific reports*, *11*(1), 1-16. https://doi.org/10.1038/s41598-021-93739-y.
5. Alligood, M. R. (2017). *Nursing theorists and their work-e-book.* 9th ED. Elsevier Health Sciences USA. P 18.
6. Alligood, M. R. (2014). *Nursing theorists and their work-e-book.* 8th ED. *Elsevier Health Sciences*. USA. P 48-50.
7. Al-Kerety, S. (2017). Effectiveness of an Education Program on Health Care Workers' Knowledge and Practices toward Infection Control at Primary Health Care Centers in Holy Kerbala City. Unpublished PhD Dissertation, University of Baghdad / College of Nursing: P. 86.

8. Al Tawil, N. G., Abdulla, M. M., & Abdul Ameer, A. J. (2007). Prevalence of and factors associated with overweight and obesity among a group of Iraqi women. *EMHJ-Eastern Mediterranean Health Journal, 13 (2), 420-429,* https://apps.who.int/iris/handle/10665/117263.
9. Al-Mudhaffer, R. H., Ahjel, S. W., Hassan, S. M., Mahmood, A. A., & Hadi, N. R. (2020). Age Distribution of Clinical Symptoms, Isolation, Co-morbidities and Case Fatality Rate of COVID-19 Cases in Najaf City, Iraq. *Medical Archives*, *74*(5),p. 365. doi: 10.5455/medarh.2020.74.363-367 .
10. Alsayed, R., Ali, A., Makia, R., Kadhom, M., Raheem, R., Al-Obaidi, O., ... & Yousif, E. (2020). Challenges Facing Iraq to Tackle the Spread of COVID-19: An Overview. *J. Uni Anbar Pure Sci*, *14*(2),p. 22.
11. Al-Tawfiq, J. A., Al-Homoud, A. H., & Memish, Z. A. (2020). Remdesivir as a possible therapeutic option for the COVID-19. *Travel medicine and infectious disease*, *34*, p.1 doi: 10.1016/j.tmaid.2020.101615.
12. Altinay, M., Sayan, I., Turk, H. S., Cinar, A. S., Sayın, P., Yucel, T., ... & Cetiner, I. (2021). Effect of early awake prone positioning application on prognosis in patients with acute respiratory failure due to COVID-19 pneumonia: a retrospective observational study. *Brazilian Journal of Anesthesiology (English Edition)*. doi.org/10.1016/j.bjane.2021.07.029
13. Altuntas, M., Yilmaz, H., and Guner, A. (2021). Evaluation of patients with COVID-19 diagnosis for chronic diseases. Virology journal, 18(1), 57. doi.org/10.1186/s12985-021-01524-0
14. Archer, S. L., Sharp, W. W., & Weir, E. K. (2020). Differentiating COVID-19 pneumonia from acute respiratory distress syndrome and

high altitude pulmonary edema: therapeutic implications. *Circulation*, *142*(2), p.103. https://doi.org/10.1161/CIRCULATIONAHA.120.047915

15. Arık, S., & Çevik, K.(2021). Effect of Postural Drainage and Deep Breathing-Cough Exercises on Oxygen Saturation, Triflo Volume and Pulmonary Function Test in Patients with COPD . Licensee Modestum. JOURNAL OF CLINICAL AND EXPERIMENTAL INVESTIGATIONS. Volume 12 • Number 4 • December 2021. em00780 .p. 1-3 https://doi.org/10.29333/jcei/11269
16. Asrani, P., Eapen, M. S., Chia, C., Haug, G., Weber, H. C., Hassan, M. I., & Sohal, S. S. (2021). Diagnostic approaches in COVID-19: clinical updates. *Expert review of respiratory medicine*, *15*(2), p.197-212. https://doi.org/10.1080/17476348.2021.1823833
17. Baj, J., Karakuła-Juchnowicz, H., Teresiński, G., Buszewicz, G., Ciesielka, M., Sitarz, E., ... & Maciejewski, R. (2020). COVID-19: specific and non-specific clinical manifestations and symptoms: the current state of knowledge. *Journal of clinical medicine*, *9*(6),p. 1753. https://doi.org/10.3390/jcm9061753
18. Bassareo, P. P., Melis, M. R., Marras, S., & Calcaterra, G. (2020). Learning from the past in the COVID-19 era: rediscovery of quarantine, previous pandemics, origin of hospitals and national healthcare systems, and ethics in medicine. *Postgraduate Medical Journal*, *96*(1140), P. 633. http://dx.doi.org/10.1136/postgradmedj-2020-138370
19. Baysal, E., MİDİLLİ, T. S., & Ergin, E. (2018). Effects of Different Position Changes on Hemodynamic Parameters and Dyspnea Severity in Patients with Dyspnea. *Clinical and Experimental Health Sciences*, *8*(4), 261-267.

20. Beeching, N. J., Fletcher, T. E., & Beadsworth, M. B. (2020). Covid-19: testing times.p. 1,2 doi: https://doi.org/10.1136/bmj.m1403
21. Behesht Aeen, F., Pakzad, R., Goudarzi Rad, M., Abdi, F., Zaheri, F., & Mirzadeh, N. (2021). Effect of prone position on respiratory parameters, intubation and death rate in COVID-19 patients: systematic review and meta-analysis. *Scientific reports*, *11*(1), 1-16. doi.org/10.1038/s41598-021-93739-y
22. Berman, A. T., Snyder, C., Frandsen, G., & Snyder, S. (2016). *Kozier & Erb's Fundamentals of Nursing, eBook, Global Eition*. Pearson Higher Ed. Chapter 50 , p. 1253
23. Bikdeli, B., Madhavan, M. V., Jimenez, D., Chuich, T., Dreyfus, I., Driggin, E., ... & Lip, G. Y. (2020). COVID-19 and thrombotic or thromboembolic disease: implications for prevention, antithrombotic therapy, and follow-up: JACC state-of-the-art review. *Journal of the American college of cardiology*, *75*(23), p.2951 doi.org/10.1016/j.jacc.2020.04.031
24. Boehmer, T. K., DeVies, J., Caruso, E., van Santen, K. L., Tang, S., Black, C. L., ... & Gundlapalli, A. V. (2020). Changing age distribution of the COVID-19 pandemic—United States, May–August 2020. *Morbidity and Mortality Weekly Report*, *69*(39), 1404 doi: 10.15585/mmwr.mm6939e1
25. Bohn, M. K., Hall, A., Sepiashvili, L., Jung, B., Steele, S., & Adeli, K. (2020). Pathophysiology of COVID-19: mechanisms underlying disease severity and progression. *Physiology*, *35*(5),p. 288. doi.org/10.1152/physiol.00019.2020
26. Brosnahan, S. B., Jonkman, A. H., Kugler, M. C., Munger, J. S., & Kaufman, D. A. (2020). COVID-19 and respiratory system disorders: current knowledge, future clinical and translational research questions. *Arteriosclerosis, thrombosis, and vascular*

biology, *40*(11), p.2586-2594. doi.org/10.1161/ATVBAHA.120.314515

27. Cai, X. F., Chen, J., li Hu, J., Long, Q. X., Deng, H. J., Liu, P., ... & Wang, D. Q. (2020). A peptide-based magnetic chemiluminescence enzyme immunoassay for serological diagnosis of coronavirus disease 2019. *The Journal of infectious diseases*, *222*(2), p. 189,193. doi.org/10.1093/infdis/jiaa243
28. Castelao, J., Graziani, D., Soriano, J., and Izquierdo, J. (2021). Findings and Prognostic Value of Lung Ultrasound in COVID-19 Pneumonia. Journal of ultrasound in medicine : official journal of the American Institute of Ultrasound in Medicine, 40(7), 1315–1324. doi.org/10.1002/jum.15508
29. Chakraborty, R., & Parvez, S. (2020). COVID-19: An overview of the current pharmacological interventions, vaccines, and clinical trials. *Biochemical pharmacology*, 114184. p. 14 doi.org/10.1016/j.bcp.2020.114184
30. Christensen, B., Favaloro, E. J., Lippi, G., & Van Cott, E. M. (2020, September). Hematology laboratory abnormalities in patients with coronavirus disease 2019 (COVID-19). In *Seminars in Thrombosis and Hemostasis*. Thieme Medical Publishers.p.1 DOI: 10.1055/s-0040-1715458
31. Coppo, A., Bellani, G., Winterton, D., Di Pierro, M., Soria, A., Faverio, P., ... & Foti, G. (2020). Feasibility and physiological effects of prone positioning in non-intubated patients with acute respiratory failure due to COVID-19 (PRON-COVID): a prospective cohort study. *The Lancet Respiratory Medicine*, *8*(8), 765-774.p. 1,2 doi.org/10.1016/S2213-2600(20)30268-X
32. Criado, P. R., Abdalla, B. M. Z., de Assis, I. C., van Blarcum de Graaff Mello, C., Caputo, G. C., & Vieira, I. C. (2020). Are the

cutaneous manifestations during or due to SARS-CoV-2 infection/COVID-19 frequent or not? Revision of possible pathophysiologic mechanisms. *Inflammation Research*, *69*,p. 747-749.
doi.org/10.1007/s00011-020-01370-w

33. Csoma, B., Vulpi, M. R., Dragonieri, S., Bentley, A., Felton, T., Lázár, Z., & Bikov, A. (2022). Hypercapnia in COPD: Causes, Consequences, and Therapy. *Journal of Clinical Medicine*, *11*(11), 3180.
34. Damarla, M., Zaeh, S., Niedermeyer, S., Merck, S., Niranjan-Azadi, A., Broderick, B., & Punjabi, N. (2020). Prone positioning of nonintubated patients with COVID-19. *American journal of respiratory and critical care medicine*, *202*(4), 604-606. doi.org/10.1164/rccm.202004-1331LE
35. Dawood, A. A., & Dawood, Z. A. (2021). How will the second wave of the dreadful COVID-19 be with the increasing number of the infected cases and mortality Iraq in? *Vacunas (English Edition)*, *22*(2), p. 118 doi.org/10.1016/j.vacune.2020.09.003
36. De Blasio, F., Virchow, J. C., Polverino, M., Zanasi, A., Behrakis, P. K., Kilinç, G., ... & Lanata, L. (2011). Cough management: a practical approach. *Cough*, *7*(1),p.1 http://www.coughjournal.com/content/7/1/7
37. Demiray, E. K. D., Çeviker, S. A., Yılmaz, M., & Alıravcı, I. D. (2021) General evaluation of the COVID 19 pandemic from an Infectious Diseases perspective.p.85 https://doi.org/10.3390/ijerph18168605
38. Dhont, S., Derom, E., Van Braeckel, E., Depuydt, P., & Lambrecht, B. N. (2020). The pathophysiology of 'happy'hypoxemia in COVID-19. *Respiratory research*, *21*(1), p.4 doi.org/10.1186/s12931-020-01462-5

39. Di Tano, G., Moschini, L., Loffi, M., Testa, S., & Danzi, G. B. (2020). Late pulmonary embolism after COVID-19 pneumonia despite adequate rivaroxaban treatment. *European Journal of Case Reports in Internal Medicine*, *7*(7).p. 2
doi: 10.12890/2020_001790

40. Dox, I. G., Melloni, B. J., Eisner, G. M., & Melloni, J. L. (2001). *Melloni's illustrated medical dictionary*. CRC Press.p.122

41. Dres, M., Goligher, E. C., Heunks, L. M., & Brochard, L. J. (2017). Critical illness-associated diaphragm weakness. *Intensive Care Medicine*, *43*(10), p.2.
DOI 10.1007/s00134-017-4928-4

42. Du, Y., Tu, L., Zhu, P., Mu, M., Wang, R., Yang, P., ... & Xu, G. (2020). Clinical features of 85 fatal cases of COVID-19 from Wuhan. A retrospective observational study. *American journal of respiratory and critical care medicine*, *201*(11), p.1376, 1377 doi.org/10.1164/rccm.202003-0543OC

43. Duong, T. A., Bouaziz, J., & Jachiet, M. M. (2020). Vascular skin symptoms in COVID-19: a french observational study. *J Eur Acad Dermatol Venereol*.p.

44. Echeverría-Esnal, D., Martin-Ontiyuelo, C., Navarrete-Rouco, M. E., De-Antonio Cuscó, M., Ferrández, O., Horcajada, J. P., & Grau, S. (2021). Azithromycin in the treatment of COVID-19: a review. *Expert Review of Anti-infective Therapy*, *19*(2), p.147 doi.org/10.1080/14787210.2020.1813024

45. Farrell, M., & Dempsey, J. (2010). *Smeltzer and Bare's textbook of medical-surgical nursing* (Vol. 2). Lippincott, Williams and Wilkins.p. 182

46. Felsenstein, S., Herbert, J. A., McNamara, P. S., & Hedrich, C. M. (2020). COVID-19: Immunology and treatment options. *Clinical immunology*, *215*, 108448.p.3 https://doi.org/10.1016/j.clim.2020.108448

47. Finzi, E. (2020). Treatment of SARS-CoV-2 with high dose oral zinc salts: A report on four patients. *International Journal of Infectious Diseases*, *99*,p. 308. https://doi.org/10.1016/j.ijid.2020.06.006

48. Fu, H., Hereward, M., MacFeely, S., Me, A., & Wilmoth, J. (2020). How COVID-19 is changing the world: A statistical perspective from the Committee for the Coordination of Statistical activities. *Statistical Journal of the IAOS*, (Preprint), p. 1-3 https://unstats.un.org/unsd/ccsa/principles_stat_activities

49. Galván Casas, C., Catala, A. C. H. G., Carretero Hernández, G., Rodríguez-Jiménez, P., Fernández-Nieto, D., Rodríguez-Villa Lario, A., ... & García-Doval, I. (2020). Classification of the cutaneous manifestations of COVID-19: a rapid prospective nationwide consensus study in Spain with 375 cases. *British Journal of Dermatology*, *183*(1), 71-77. https://doi.org/10.1111/bjd.19163

50. Garcia, L. P. R. D. R., Abreu, C. C. S., Abe, A. H. D. M., & Matos, M. A. D. (2021). Reflections on passive smoking and COVID-19. *Revista da Associação Médica Brasileira*, *67*, 22-25.

51. Gartner-Schmidt, J. L., Shembel, A. C., Zullo, T. G., & Rosen, C. A. (2014). Development and validation of the Dyspnea Index (DI): a severity index for upper airway–related dyspnea. *Journal of Voice*, *28*(6),P. 778 https://doi.org/10.1016/j.jvoice.2013.12.017

52. Gattinoni, L., Chiumello, D., & Rossi, S. (2020). COVID-19 pneumonia: ARDS or not?. *Critical care*, *24*(1), 1-3. https://doi.org/10.1186/s13054-020-02880-z
53. Gattinoni, L., Chiumello, D., Caironi, P., Busana, M., Romitti, F., Brazzi, L., & Camporota, L. (2020). COVID-19 pneumonia: different respiratory treatments for different phenotypes p.2, 1099,1100 https://doi.org/10.1007/s00134-020-06033-2
54. George, P. M., Barratt, S. L., Condliffe, R., Desai, S. R., Devaraj, A., Forrest, I., ... & Spencer, L. G. (2020). Respiratory follow-up of patients with COVID-19 pneumonia. *Thorax*, *75*(11), p.1012 http://thorax.bmj.com
55. Gray, J. R., Grove, S. K., & Sutherland, S. (2016). Burns and grove's the practice of nursing research-E-book: Appraisal, synthesis, and generation of evidence. Elsevier Health Sciences.p. 534
56. Henderson, W. R., Griesdale, D. E., Dominelli, P., & Ronco, J. J. (2014). Does prone positioning improve oxygenation and reduce mortality in patients with acute respiratory distress syndrome?. *Canadian respiratory journal*, *21*(4), 213-215. https://doi.org/10.1155/2014/472136
57. Hendren, N. S., de Lemos, J. A., Ayers, C., Das, S. R., Rao, A., Carter, S., ... & Grodin, J. L. (2021). Association of body mass index and age with morbidity and mortality in patients hospitalized with COVID-19: results from the American Heart Association COVID-19 Cardiovascular Disease Registry. *Circulation*, *143*(2), 135-144. https://doi.org/10.1161/CIRCULATIONAHA.120.051936
58. Hughes, S. J. (2022). Kozier and Erb's Fundamentals of Nursing: Concepts, Process and Practice, A. Berman, S. Snyder (Eds.), ELEVEN EDITION, –International ed., Pearson, Boston (2022)[Book Review]. *Nurse Education in Practice*, *12*(2), e12.

59. Ibraheem, M. K., Abedalrahman, S. K., Sarhat, A. R., & Al-Diwan, J. K. (2021). Prone positioning is helpful in management of wake spontaneously breathing COVID 19 patients. *Dokkyo Journal of Medical Sciences*, *48*(02), p. 55.
60. Imamoğlu, O., & Dilek, A. N. (2016). Common benefits of prayer and yoga on human organism. *International Journal of Sport Culture and Science*, *4*(Special Issue 2), 639-651.
61. Jarosz, O. A., Szmelcer, B., & Podhorecka, M. (2020). Application and effectiveness of respiratory physiotherapy in the prevention and treatment of patients with Covid-19. *Medical Research Journal*, *5*(4), 265-270.
http://www.journals.viamedica.pl/medical_research_journal
62. Jin, P., Park, H., Jung, S., & Kim, J. (2021). Challenges in Urology during the COVID-19 Pandemic. *Urologia internationalis*, *105*(1-2), P.9-16.
https://doi.org/10.1159/000512880
63. Joshi, S., Parkar, J., Ansari, A., Vora, A., Talwar, D., Tiwaskar, M., ... & Barkate, H. (2020). Role of favipiravir in the treatment of COVID-19. *International Journal of Infectious Diseases*. https://doi.org/10.1016/j.ijid.2020.10.069
64. Kako, J., Morita, T., Yamaguchi, T., Kobayashi, M., Sekimoto, A., Kinoshita, H., ... & Matsushima, E. (2018). Fan therapy is effective in relieving dyspnea in patients with terminally ill cancer: a Parallel-Arm, randomized controlled trial. *Journal of pain and symptom management*, *56*(4), p.2
https://doi.org/10.1016/j.jpainsymman.2018.07.001
65. Kwok, S., Adam, S., Ho, J. H., Iqbal, Z., Turkington, P., Razvi, S., ... & Syed, A. A. (2020). Obesity: a critical risk factor in the COVID-

19 pandemic. *Clinical obesity*, *10*(6), e12403. https://doi.org/10.1111/cob.12403

66. Kwong, J. C., Schwartz, K. L., Campitelli, M. A., Chung, H., Crowcroft, N. S., Karnauchow, T., ... & Gubbay, J. B. (2018). Acute myocardial infarction after laboratory-confirmed influenza infection. *New England Journal of Medicine*, *378*(4), p. 346 DOI: 10.1056/NEJMoa1702090
67. Lahiri, D., & Ardila, A. (2020). COVID-19 pandemic: a neurological perspective. *Cureus*, *12*(4).p.1-4 DOI: 10.7759/cureus.7889
68. Lai, C. C., Shih, T. P., Ko, W. C., Tang, H. J., & Hsueh, P. R. (2020). Severe acute respiratory syndrome coronavirus 2 (SARS-CoV-2) and coronavirus disease-2019 (COVID-19): The pandemic and the challenges. *International journal of antimicrobial agents*, *55*(3), 105924.p.3. https://doi.org/10.1016/j.ijantimicag.2020.105924
69. Langer, T., Brioni, M., Guzzardella, A., Carlesso, E., Cabrini, L., Castelli, G., ... & Grasselli, G. (2021). Prone position in intubated, mechanically ventilated patients with COVID-19: a multi-centric study of more than 1000 patients. *Critical Care*, *25*(1), p.1. https://doi.org/10.1186/s13054-021-03552-2
70. Lee, S., Lasky-Su, J. A., Lange, C., Kim, W., Kumar, P. L., McDonald, M. L. N., ... & Hecker, J. (2021). A novel locus for exertional dyspnoea in childhood asthma. *European Respiratory Journal*, *57*(2). DOI: 10.1183/13993003.01224-2020
71. Lee, S., Son, K., Han, C., Jung, J., & and Park, S. (2020). Impact of comorbid asthma on severity of coronavirus disease (COVID-19). *Scientific reports*, *10*(1), 1-9. https://doi.org/10.1038/s41598-020-77791-8

72. Levi, M., & Thachil, J. (2020, October). Coronavirus Disease 2019 Coagulopathy: Disseminated Intravascular Coagulation and Thrombotic Microangiopathy—Either, Neither, or Both. In *Seminars in thrombosis and hemostasis* (Vol. 46, No. 07, pp. 781-784). DOI: 10.1055/s-0040-1712156

73. Li, H., Zhao, Y., Zhou, L., & Hu, J. (2020). Cutaneous, skin histopathological manifestations and relationship to COVID-19 infection patients. *Dermatologic therapy*, *33*(6), P.3 https://doi.org/10.1111/dth.14157

74. Lippi, G., Wong, J., & Henry, B. M. (2020). Hypertension and its severity or mortality in Coronavirus Disease 2019 (COVID-19): a pooled analysis. *Pol Arch Intern Med*, *130*(4), p. 307.

75. Liu, K., Chen, Y., Lin, R., & Han, K. (2020). Clinical features of COVID-19 in elderly patients: A comparison with young and middle-aged patients. *Journal of Infection*, *80*(6), e14-e18.p.16 https://doi.org/10.1016/j.jinf.2020.03.005

76. Long, B., Brady, W. J., Koyfman, A., & Gottlieb, M. (2020). Cardiovascular complications in COVID-19. *The American journal of emergency medicine*, *38*(7), 1504-1507 https://doi.org/10.1016/j.ajem.2020.04.048

77. Mahrous, E. S., & Aboelmagd, A. (2022). Effect of knee-chest, semi-sitting, and right lateral position on preterm neonates with respiratory distress syndrome. *International Egyptian Journal of Nursing Sciences and Research*, *2*(2), 353-361.
DOI: 10.21608/ejnsr.2022.212952

78. Mangal, A., Kalia, S., Rajgopal, H., Rangarajan, K., Namboodiri, V., Banerjee, S., & Arora, C. (2020). CovidAID: COVID-19 detection using chest X-ray. *P.3,4* https://doi.org/10.48550/arXiv.2004.09803

79. Marik, P., DePerrior, S., Ahmad, Q., and Dodani. S. (2021). Gender-based Disparities in COVID-19 Patient Outcomes. Journal of Investigative Medicine. 69:814-818. Retrieved from https://jim.bmj.com/content/69/4/814.info

80. Matschke, J., Lütgehetmann, M., Hagel, C., Sperhake, J. P., Schröder, A. S., Edler, C., ... & Glatzel, M. (2020). Neuropathology of patients with COVID-19 in Germany: a post-mortem case series. *The Lancet Neurology*, *19*(11), p.1,2 https://doi.org/10.1016/S1474-4422(20)30308-2

81. McNicholas, B., Cosgrave, D., Giacomini, C., Brennan, A., & Laffey, J. G. (2020). Prone positioning in COVID-19 acute respiratory failure: just do it?. *BJA: British Journal of Anaesthesia*, *125*(4), 440. doi: 10.1016/j.bja.2020.06.003

82. Mehta, J. L., Calcaterra, G., & Bassareo, P. P. (2020). COVID-19, thromboembolic risk, and Virchow's triad: Lesson from the past. *Clinical Cardiology*, *43*(12), p. 1364 https://doi.org/10.1002/clc.23460

83. Ministry of Health / Environment / Public Health Department. 2022. The daily epidemiological and vaccination situation of the Corona pandemic in Iraq, March 1, 2022. www.facebook.com/MOH.GOV.IQ

84. Moghadam, V. D., Shafiee, H., Ghorbani, M., & Heidarifar, R. (2020). Prone positioning in management of COVID-19 hospitalized patients. *Revista Brasileira de Anestesiologia*, *70*, 188-188. doi.org/10.1016/j.bjane.2020.05.001

85. Mohammadi, M., Khamseh, A. K. P., & Varpaei, H. A. (2021). Invasive Airway" Intubation" in COVID-19 Patients; Statistics, Causes, and Recommendations: A Review Article. *Anesthesiology and Pain Medicine*, *11*(3). doi: 10.5812/aapm.115868

86. Morens, D. M., Daszak, P., Markel, H., & Taubenberger, J. K. (2020). Pandemic COVID-19 joins history's pandemic legion. *MBio*, *11*(3), p.1

87. Mueller, A. L., McNamara, M. S., & Sinclair, D. A. (2020). Why does COVID-19 disproportionately affect older people?. *Aging (albany NY)*, *12*(10), 9959.
doi: 10.18632/aging.103344

88. Munro, B. H. (2005). *Statistical methods for health care research* (Vol. 1). lippincott williams & wilkins.p. 395

89. Henning, R. J., Feliciano, L., & Coers, C. M. (1996). Vagal nerve stimulation increases right ventricular contraction and relaxation and heart rate. *Cardiovascular Research*, *32*(5), 846-853.

90. Nieswiadomy, R. (2012). Foundations of Nursing Research. 6th Edition. Pearson Education, USA: 122

91. Niikawa, H., Okamoto, T., Ayyat, K. S., Itoda, Y., Farver, C. F., & McCurry, K. R. (2019). The protective effect of prone lung position on ischemia–reperfusion injury and lung function in an ex vivo porcine lung model. *The Journal of thoracic and cardiovascular surgery*, *157*(1), 425-433. https://doi.org/10.1016/j.jtcvs.2018.08.101

92. Nolt, B. R., Gonzales, R., Maselli, J., Aagaard, E., Camargo Jr, C. A., & Metlay, J. P. (2007). Vital-sign abnormalities as predictors of pneumonia in adults with acute cough illness. *The American journal of emergency medicine*, *25*(6), 631-636. https://doi.org/10.1016/j.ajem.2006.11.031

93. Nouchi, A., Chastang, J., Miyara, M., Lejeune, J., Soares, A., Ibanez, G., ... & Pourcher, V. (2021). Prevalence of hyposmia and hypogeusia in 390 COVID-19 hospitalized patients and outpatients: a cross-sectional study. *European Journal of Clinical Microbiology*

& Infectious Diseases, *40*(4),p. 691 https://doi.org/10.1007/s10096-020-04056-7

94. Ora, J., Liguori, C., Puxeddu, E., Coppola, A., Matino, M., Pierantozzi, M., ... & Rogliani, P. (2020). Dyspnea perception and neurological symptoms in non-severe COVID-19 patients. *Neurological Sciences*, *41*(10), p. 2671 https://doi.org/10.1007/s10072-020-04632-x
95. Orsucci, D., Ienco, E. C., Nocita, G., Napolitano, A., & Vista, M. (2020). Neurological features of COVID-19 and their treatment: a review. *Drugs in context*, *9*.p. 1-3 doi: 10.7573/dic.2020-5-1
96. Osinibi, M., Gupta, A., Harman, K., and Bossley, C. (2021). Passive tobacco smoke in children and young people during the COVID-19 pandemic. The Lancet. Respiratory medicine, 9(7), 693–694. https://doi.org/10.1016/S2213-2600(21)00231-9
97. Pan, L., Mu, M., Yang, P., Sun, Y., Wang, R., Yan, J., ... & Tu, L. (2020). Clinical characteristics of COVID-19 patients with digestive symptoms in Hubei, China: a descriptive, cross-sectional, multicenter study. *The American journal of gastroenterology*, *115*. p.770 doi: 10.14309/ajg.0000000000000620
98. Patanavanich, R., and Glantz, S. (2021). Smoking is associated with worse outcomes of COVID-19 particularly among younger adults: a systematic review and meta-analysis. BMC Public Health. 21:1554 https://doi.org/10.1186/s12889-021-11579-x
99. Pereira, A. A., de Oliveira Andrade, A., de Andrade Palis, A., Cabral, A. M., Barreto, C. G. L., de Souza, D. B., ... & da Conceição Lima, V. (2021). Non-pharmacological treatments for COVID-19: current status and consensus. *Research on Biomedical Engineering*, P.1-16. https://doi.org/10.1007/s42600-020-00116-1

100. Petersen, E., Ntoumi, F., Hui, D. S., Abubakar, A., Kramer, L. D., Obiero, C., ... & Zumla, A. (2022). Emergence of new SARS-CoV-2 Variant of Concern Omicron (B. 1.1. 529)-highlights Africa's research capabilities, but exposes major knowledge gaps, inequities of vaccine distribution, inadequacies in global COVID-19 response and control efforts. *International Journal of Infectious Diseases*, *114*, 268-272. https://doi.org/10.1016/j.ijid.2021.11.040

101. Pola, A., Murthy, K. S., & Santhekadur, P. K. (2021). COVID-19 and gastrointestinal system: A brief review. *Biomedical Journal*.p. 246-250 https://doi.org/10.1016/j.bj.2021.01.001

102. Pranata, R., Lim, M. A., Huang, I., Raharjo, S. B., & Lukito, A. A. (2020). Hypertension is associated with increased mortality and severity of disease in COVID-19 pneumonia: a systematic review, meta-analysis and meta-regression. *Journal of the renin-angiotensin-aldosterone system: JRAAS*, *21*(2).p.1 doi: 10.1177/1470320320926899

103. Priyadarshini, (2021). Lydia E. Hall Theory, Core, Care and Cure Model, IJRTI | Volume 6, Issue 9 | ISSN: 2456-3315

104. Raisi-Estabragh, Z., McCracken, C., Ardissino, M., Bethell, M., Cooper, J., Cooper, C., ... and Petersen, S. (2020). Non-white ethnicity, male sex, and higher body mass index, but not medications acting on the renin-angiotensin system are associated with coronavirus disease 2019 (COVID-19) hospitalisation: review of the first 669 cases from the UK Biobank. *MedRxiv*. https://doi.org/10.1101/2020.05.10.20096925

105. Recalcati, S. Cutaneous manifestations in COVID-19: a first perspective [published online March 26, 2020]. *J Eur Acad Dermatol Venereol. doi*, *10*.p. 3

106. Retucci, M., Aliberti, S., Ceruti, C., Santambrogio, M., Tammaro, S., Cuccarini, F., ... & Blasi, F. (2020). Prone and lateral positioning in spontaneously breathing patients with COVID-19 pneumonia undergoing noninvasive helmet CPAP treatment. *Chest*, *158*(6), 2431.p.2,3. https://doi.org/10.1016/j.chest.2020.07.006

107. Rizk, J. G., Gupta, A., Sardar, P., Henry, B. M., Lewin, J. C., Lippi, G., & Lavie, C. J. (2021). Clinical Characteristics and Pharmacological Management of COVID-19 Vaccine–Induced Immune Thrombotic Thrombocytopenia with Cerebral Venous Sinus Thrombosis: A Review. *JAMA cardiology*.p.6 doi:10.1001/jamacardio.2021.3444

108. Rogero, M. M., Leão, M. D. C., Santana, T. M., de MB Pimentel, M. V., Carlini, G. C., da Silveira, T. F., ... & Castro, I. A. (2020). Potential benefits and risks of omega-3 fatty acids supplementation to patients with COVID-19. *Free Radical Biology and Medicine*.P. 194,195 https://doi.org/10.1016/j.freeradbiomed.2020.07.005

109. Sachs, J. D., Horton, R., Bagenal, J., Amor, Y. B., Caman, O. K., & Lafortune, G. (2020). The lancet COVID-19 commission. *The Lancet*, *396*(10249), 454-455.p.2 DOI:https://doi.org/10.1016/S0140-6736(20)31927-9

110. Salim, A. I. M. A. (2021). Prostration Utterances in the Glorious Qur'an; A linguistic Study. *Journal of Language Studies*, *4*(1), p.17

111. Sartini, C., Tresoldi, M., Scarpellini, P., Tettamanti, A., Carcò, F., Landoni, G., & Zangrillo, A. (2020). Respiratory parameters in patients with COVID-19 after using noninvasive ventilation in the prone position outside the intensive care unit. *Jama*, *323*(22), 2338-2340. doi:10.1001/jama.2020.7861

112. Seneviwickrama, M., Kantharuban, D., Rodrigo, C., Karunarathna, B., Talagala, I., Gunatilake, I., ... & Goonewardena, S. (2020).

COVID-19: the first coronavirus pandemic. *Journal of the College of Community Physicians of Sri Lanka*, *26*(5).p. 1-4

113. Sestili, P., & Fimognari, C. (2020). Paracetamol-induced glutathione consumption: is there a link with severe COVID-19 illness?. *Frontiers in pharmacology*, *11*, 1597. p. 2 https://doi.org/10.3389/fphar.2020.579944

114. Shah, V., Keniya, R., Shridharani, A., Punjabi, M., Shah, J., & Mehendale, N. (2021). Diagnosis of COVID-19 using CT scan images and deep learning techniques. *Emergency radiology*, *28*(3), p.498 https://doi.org/10.1007/s10140-020-01886-y

115. Shakoor, H., Feehan, J., Al Dhaheri, A. S., Ali, H. I., Platat, C., Ismail, L. C., ... & Stojanovska, L. (2021). Immune-boosting role of vitamins D, C, E, zinc, selenium and omega-3 fatty acids: Could they help against COVID-19?. *Maturitas*, *143*, p.1-16. https://doi.org/10.1016/j.maturitas.2020.08.003

116. Shembel, A. C., Rosen, C. A., Zullo, T. G., & Gartner-Schmidt, J. L. (2013). Development and validation of the cough severity index: a severity index for chronic cough related to the upper airway. *The Laryngoscope*, *123*(8), p. 1934. https://doi.org/10.1002/lary.23916

117. Sheraton, M., Deo, N., Kashyap, R., & Surani, S. (2020). A review of neurological complications of COVID-19. *Cureus*, *12*(5).P.5 doi:10.7759/cureus.8192

118. Singh, R., Kang, A., Luo, X., Jeyanathan, M., Gillgrass, A., Afkhami, S., & Xing, Z. (2021). COVID-19: Current knowledge in clinical features, immunological responses, and vaccine development. *The FASEB Journal*, *35*(3), e21409.p.3 https://doi.org/10.1096/fj.202002662R

119. Singhal, T. (2020). A review of coronavirus disease-2019 (COVID-19). *The indian journal of pediatrics*, *87*(4), p.285

120. Slessarev, M., Cheng, J., Ondrejicka, M., & Arntfield, R. (2020). Patient self-proning with high-flow nasal cannula improves oxygenation in COVID-19 pneumonia. *Canadian Journal of Anesthesia/Journal canadien d'anesthésie*, *67*(9), 1288-1290.p.1 https://doi.org/10.1007/s12630-020-01661-0

121. Smith, K., Warner, P., Williams, L. J., Adamson, W. E., Katikireddi, S. V., Dewart, P., ... & Mackenzie, D. G. (2011). Prevalence of influenza A (H1N1) seropositivity in unvaccinated healthcare workers in Scotland at the height of the global pandemic. *Journal of environmental and public health*, *2011*.p. 1,2 https://doi.org/10.1155/2011/407505

122. Smith, M. C. (2010). Nursing theories and nursing practice. FA Davis, 3rd ed. Philadelphia, PA 19103. USA, ISO 690 P. 54-64.

123. Soldati, G., Smargiassi, A., Inchingolo, R., Buonsenso, D., Perrone, T., Briganti, D., Perlini, S., Torri, E., Mariani, A., Mossolani, E., Tursi, F., Mento, F., and Demi, L. (2020). Is There a Role for Lung Ultrasound During the COVID-19 Pandemic?. Journal of ultrasound in medicine : official journal of the American Institute of Ultrasound in Medicine, 39(7), 1459–1462. https://doi.org/10.1002/jum.15284

124. Song, W. J., Hui, C. K., Hull, J. H., Birring, S. S., McGarvey, L., Mazzone, S. B., & Chung, K. F. (2021). Confronting COVID-19-associated cough and the post-COVID syndrome: role of viral neurotropism, neuroinflammation, and neuroimmune responses. *The Lancet Respiratory Medicine*.p. 533-538 https://doi.org/10.1016/S2213-2600(21)00125-9

125. South, A. M., Diz, D. I., & Chappell, M. C. (2020). COVID-19, ACE2, and the cardiovascular consequences. *American Journal of Physiology-Heart and Circulatory Physiology*, *318*(5), p. 1084, 1085 https://doi.org/10.1152/ajpheart.00217.2020

126. Struyf, T., Deeks, J. J., Dinnes, J., Takwoingi, Y., Davenport, C., Leeflang, M. M., ... & COVID, C. (2021). Signs and symptoms to determine if a patient presenting in primary care or hospital outpatient settings has COVID-19. *Cochrane Database of Systematic Reviews*, (2).p .1-9 https://doi.org/10.1002/14651858.CD013665.pub2

127. Sumarno, A. S. (2019). Pressure ulcers: the core, care and cure approach. British Journal of Community Nursing, 24(Sup12), S38-S42. https://doi.org/10.12968/bjcn.2019.24.Sup12.S38

128. Sun, Y., Dong, Y., Wang, L., Xie, H., Li, B., Chang, C., & Wang, F. S. (2020). Characteristics and prognostic factors of disease severity in patients with COVID-19: The Beijing experience. *Journal of autoimmunity*, *112*, 102473. https://doi.org/10.1016/j.jaut.2020.102473

129. Suwanwongse, K., & Shabarek, N. (2020). Hyperpyrexia in patients with COVID-19. *Journal of medical virology*, *92*(11),p. 2857-2859 https://doi.org/10.1002/jmv.26154

130. Swenson, K. E., Ruoss, S. J., & Swenson, E. R. (2021). The pathophysiology and dangers of silent hypoxemia in COVID-19 lung injury. *Annals of the American Thoracic Society*, (ja).p. 1098 https://doi.org/10.1513/AnnalsATS.202011-1376CME

131. Tahamtan, A., & Ardebili, A. (2020). Real-time RT-PCR in COVID-19 detection: issues affecting the results. *Expert review of molecular diagnostics*, *20*(5), p. 453-454. https://doi.org/10.1080/14737159.2020.1757437

132. Thompson, A. E., Ranard, B. L., Wei, Y., & Jelic, S. (2020). Prone positioning in awake, nonintubated patients with COVID-19 hypoxemic respiratory failure. *JAMA internal medicine*, *180*(11), p.1537-1539. doi:10.1001/jamainternmed.2020.3030

133. Tobaiqy, M., Qashqary, M., Al-Dahery, S., Mujallad, A., Hershan, A. A., Kamal, M. A., & Helmi, N. (2020). Therapeutic management of patients with COVID-19: a systematic review. *Infection Prevention in Practice*, *2*(3), p.1 https://doi.org/10.1016/j.infpip.2020.100061

134. Touchon, F., Trigui, Y., Prud'homme, E., Lefebvre, L., Giraud, A., Dols, A., Martinez, S., Bernardi, M., Begne, C., Granier, P., Chanez, P., Forel, J., Papazian, L., and Elharrar, X. (2021). Awake prone positioning for hypoxaemic respiratory failure: past, COVID-19 and perspectives. European respiratory Review: an official journal of the European Respiratory Society, 30(160), 210022. https://doi.org/10.1183/16000617.0022-2021

135. Umara, A. F. (2018). THE MODEL THEORY APPROACH" CARE, CORE, CURU" FOR PATIENTS WITH CARDIOVASCULAR DISEASES. International Journal of Nursing and Health Services (IJNHS), 1(2), 120-128.p.6,7 https://doi.org/10.35654/ijnhs.v1i2.53

136. Urme, N. A., Alam, F., & Rahman, E. (2019). Effectiveness of Active Cycle of Breathing Technique (ACBT) for the Patients of Bronchiectasis: A Narrative Review Study. *J Clin Respir Dis Care*, *5*(142),.p.2

137. Vardavas, C. I., & Nikitara, K. (2020). COVID-19 and smoking: A systematic review of the evidence. *Tobacco induced diseases*, *18*. doi: 10.18332/tid/119324

138. Venus, K., Munshi, L., & Fralick, M. (2020). Prone positioning for patients with hypoxic respiratory failure related to COVID-19. *Cmaj*, *192*(47), E1532-E1537.

139. Wang, H. Y., Li, X. L., Yan, Z. R., Sun, X. P., Han, J., & Zhang, B. W. (2020). Potential neurological symptoms of COVID-

19. *Therapeutic advances in neurological disorders*, *p.1* https://doi.org/10.1503/cmaj.201201

140. Wang, M., Cao, R., Zhang, L., Yang, X., Liu, J., Xu, M., ... & Xiao, G. (2020). Remdesivir and chloroquine effectively inhibit the recently emerged novel coronavirus (2019-nCoV) in vitro. *Cell research*, *30*(3), p.26 https://doi.org/10.1038/s41422-020-0282-0

141. Williams, L. S., & Hopper, P. D. (2015). *Understanding medical surgical nursing*. FA Davis.p.608

142. Wilson, M. H., Edsell, M. E., Davagnanam, I., Hirani, S. P., Martin, D. S., Levett, D. Z., ... & Caudwell Xtreme Everest Research Group. (2011). Cerebral artery dilatation maintains cerebral oxygenation at extreme altitude and in acute hypoxia—an ultrasound and MRI study. *Journal of Cerebral Blood Flow & Metabolism*, *31*(10), 2019-2029.

143. Wollina, U., Karadağ, A. S., Rowland-Payne, C., Chiriac, A., & Lotti, T. (2020). Cutaneous signs in COVID-19 patients: a review. *Dermatologic therapy*, *33*(5), p. 1-6 https://doi.org/10.1111/dth.13549

144. World Health Organization. (2020). *Clinical management of COVID-19: interim guidance, 27 May 2020* (No. WHO/2019-nCoV/clinical/2020.5). World Health Organization.p.2. https:// WHO/2019-nCoV/clinical/2020.5

145. World Health Organization. (2022). COVID-19 weekly epidemiological update, edition 80, 22 February 2022. https://apps.who.int/iris/handle/10665/352199

146. Wu, S. C. (2020). Progress and concept for COVID-19 vaccine development. *Biotechnology journal*.p. 1 doi: 10.1002/biot.202000147

147. Wu, Z. S., Zhang, Z. Q., & Wu, S. (2020). Focus on the crosstalk between COVID-19 and urogenital systems.p. 7 https://doi.org/10.1097/JU.0000000000001068

148. Xie, J., Covassin, N., Fan, Z., Singh, P., Gao, W., Li, G. & Somers, V. K. (2020, June). Association between hypoxemia and mortality in patients with COVID-19. In *Mayo Clinic Proceedings* (Vol. 95, No. 6, pp. 1138-1147). Elsevier.p. 1138 https://doi.org/10.1016/j.mayocp.2020.04.006

149. Ye, G., Pan, Z., Pan, Y., Deng, Q., Chen, L., Li, J., ... & Wang, X. (2020). Clinical characteristics of severe acute respiratory syndrome coronavirus 2 reactivation. *Journal of Infection*, *80*(5), e14-e17.p. 2,3 https://doi.org/10.1016/j.jinf.2020.03.001

150. Yusoff, M. S. B. (2019). ABC of content validation and content validity index calculation. *Resource*, *11*(2), 49-54. https://doi.org/10.21315/eimj2019.11.2.6

151. Yusoff, M. S. B. (2019). ABC of response process validation and face validity index calculation. *Resource*, *11*(3). https://doi.org/10.21315/eimj2019.11.3.6

152. Yuan, H., & Silberstein, S. D. (2016). Vagus nerve and vagus nerve stimulation, a comprehensive review: part I. *Headache: The Journal of Head and Face Pain*, *56*(1), 71-78.

153. Zang, X., Wang, Q., Zhou, H., Liu, S., & Xue, X. (2020). Efficacy of early prone position for COVID-19 patients with severe hypoxia: a single-center prospective cohort study. *Intensive care medicine*, *46*(10), p. 1927 https://doi.org/10.1007/s00134-020-06182-4

154. Zhang, H., & Baker, A. (2017). Recombinant human ACE2: acing out angiotensin II in ARDS therapy.p.1 DOI 10.1186/s13054-017-1882-z

155. Zhang, P., Qu, Y., Tu, J., Cao, W., Hai, N., Li, S., ... & Guo, R. (2020). Applicability of bedside ultrasonography for the diagnosis of deep venous thrombosis in patients with COVID-19 and treatment with low molecular weight heparin. *Journal of Clinical Ultrasound*, *48*(9),p. 522,523. https://doi.org/10.1002/jcu.22898

156. Zhou, Y., Fu, B., Zheng, X., Wang, D., Zhao, C., Sun, R., ... & Wei, H. (2020). Aberrant pathogenic GM-CSF+ T cells and inflammatory CD14+ CD16+ monocytes in severe pulmonary syndrome patients of a new coronavirus. *BioRxiv*.p.1 doi: https://doi.org/10.1101/2020.02.12.945576

157. Zhu, J., Ji, P., Pang, J., Zhong, Z., Li, H., He, C., ... & Zhao, C. (2020). Clinical characteristics of 3062 COVID-19 patients: a meta-analysis. *Journal of medical virology*, *92*(10), p.1902. https://doi.org/10.1002/jmv.25884

Appendices

Applying prostrate position

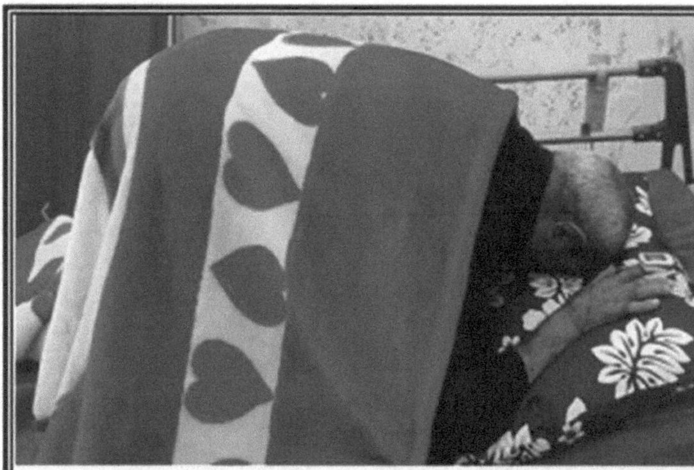

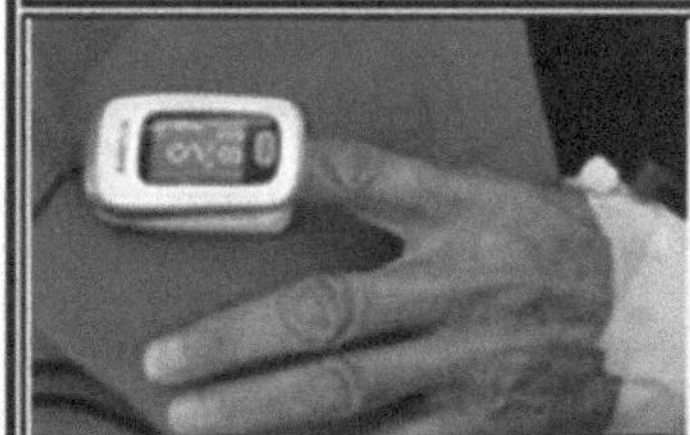

Picture (1) PR and SPO2 Before performing the prostrate position

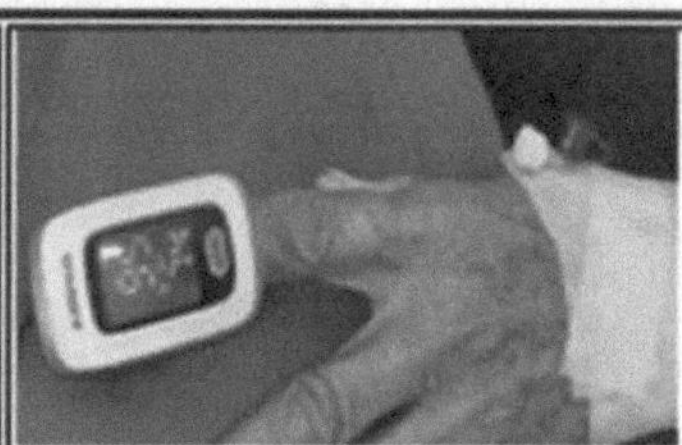

Picture (2) PR and SPO2 After a full hour of performing the prostrate position

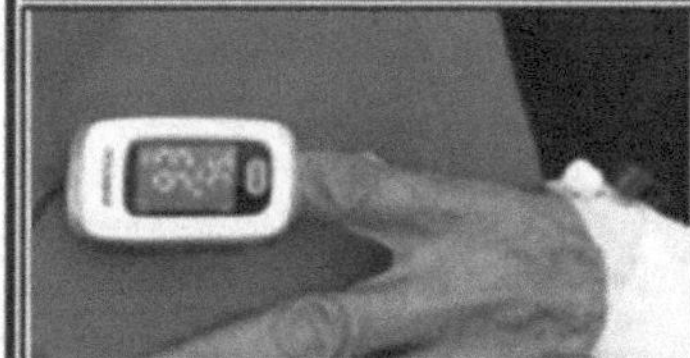

Picture (3) PR and SPO2 After 4 hours from performing the prostrate position

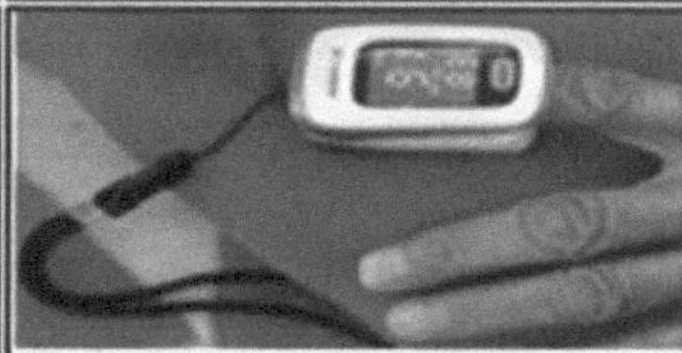

Picture (4) PR and SPO2 After 7 hours from performing the prostration position

Applying prostrate position

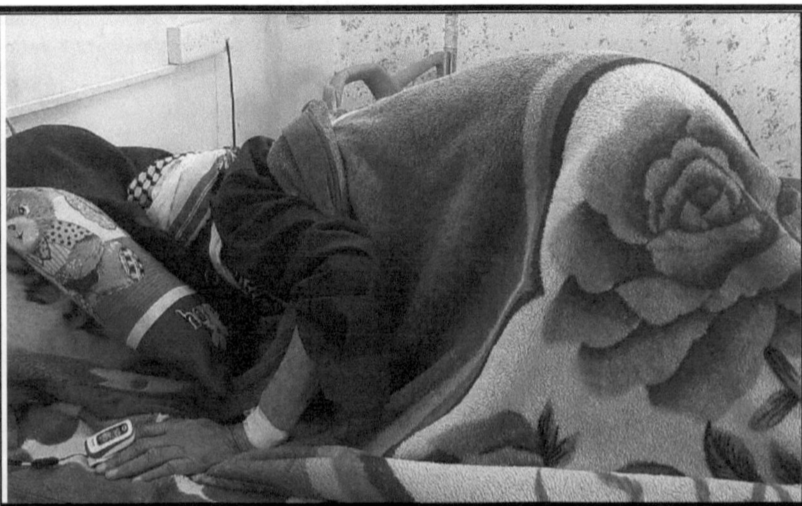

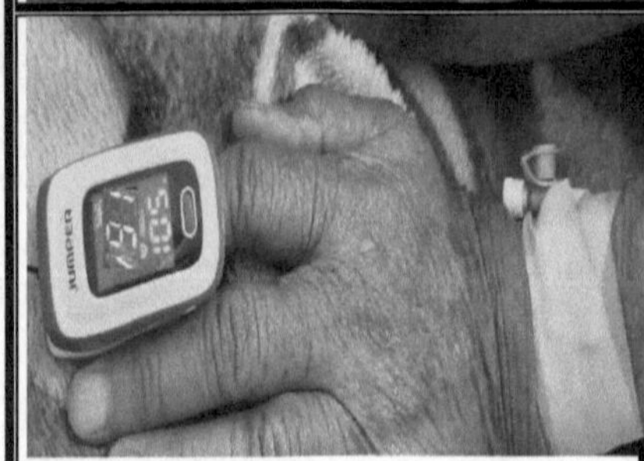

Picture (1) PR and SPO2 Before performing the prostrate position

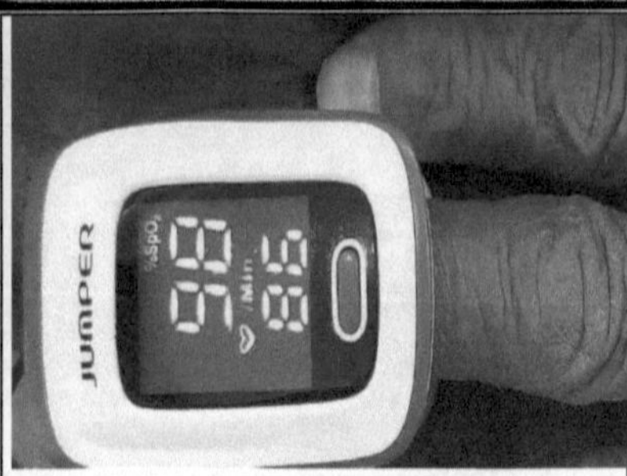

Picture (2) PR and SPO2 After a full hour of performing the prostrate position

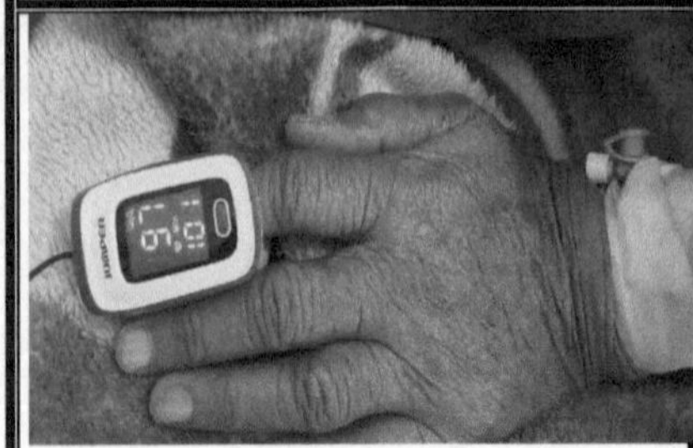

Picture (3) PR and SPO2 After 4 hours from performing the prostrate position

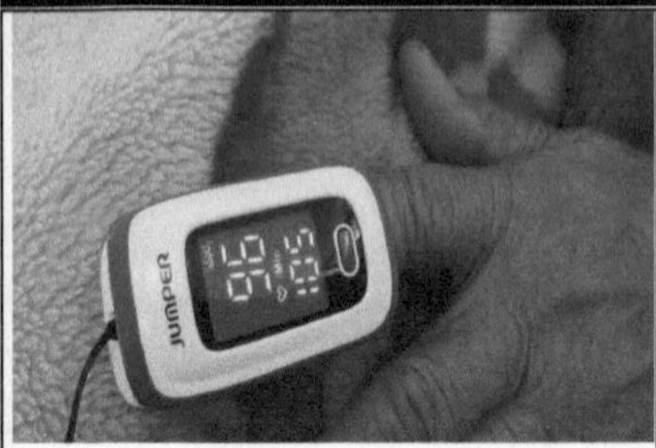

Picture (4) PR and SPO2 After 7 hours from performing the prostration position

Applying coughing exercises

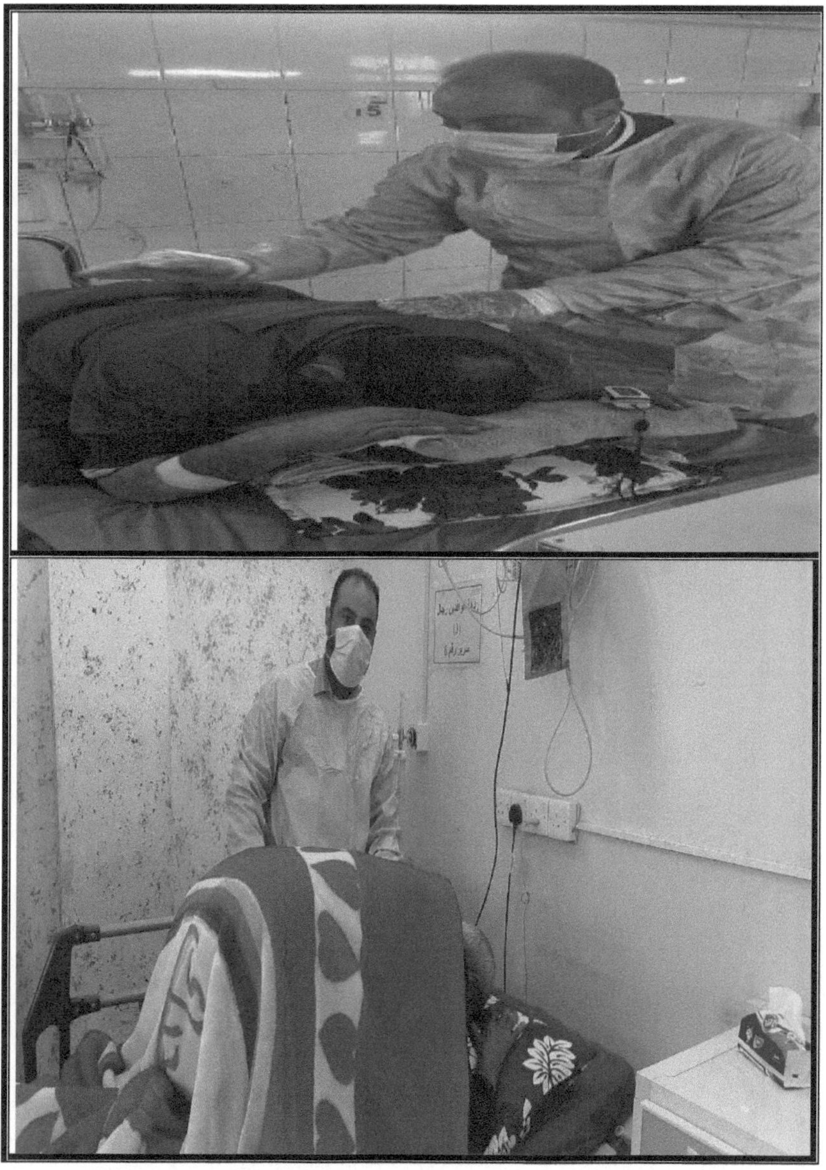

موافقة خطية للمشاركة بالبحث

موافقة خطية للمشاركة في بحث

الرجاء التوقيع أسفل الصفحة كي تشهد بان:

بعد أن قام طالب الماجستير **(حيدر نواف عبد علي)** بشرح وتوضيح جميع التساؤلات بخصوص بحثه الموسوم (اثر وضع السجود وتمارين السعال في مستوى ضيق التنفس، السعال المستمر، والمؤشرات القلبة -الرئوية بين المرضى غير المنبوبين المصابين بفيروس كورونا 19)، حيث أطلعني صاحب البحث عن فائدة بحثه وأهميته العلمية .كما وأطلعني بان مشاركتي هذه هي تطوع مني وبمحض إرادتي و أن باستطاعتي رفض المُشاركة كما أن بإمكاني سحب مشاركتي في الدراسة متى شئت ولأي سبب كان ، او ان لا اجيب على أي سؤال لا ارغب في إجابته، كما تم إعلامي بان مشاركتي بالبحث لن تحملني أي نفقات أو مسائلة من شانها الضرر بمهنتي أو شخصيتي، كما إن المعلومات الناتجة عن مشاركتي سوف تعامل بسرية تامة ولن يطلع عليها أي شخص وان هذه المعلومات ونتائجها هي للأغراض العلمية فقط ولن تكون هناك أي إشارة إلى شخصي أو عائلتي في أي منشور عن هذه الدراسة.

ولأجل هذا فاني أوقع على مشاركتي في هذا البحث

يرجى كتابة التاريخ بجانب التوقيع

توقيع المشارك .... التاريخ ٢٦ / ١ / ٢٠٢٢

توقيع الباحث .... التاريخ ٢٦ / ١ / ٢٠٢٢

TABLE DES MATIÈRES

More Books!

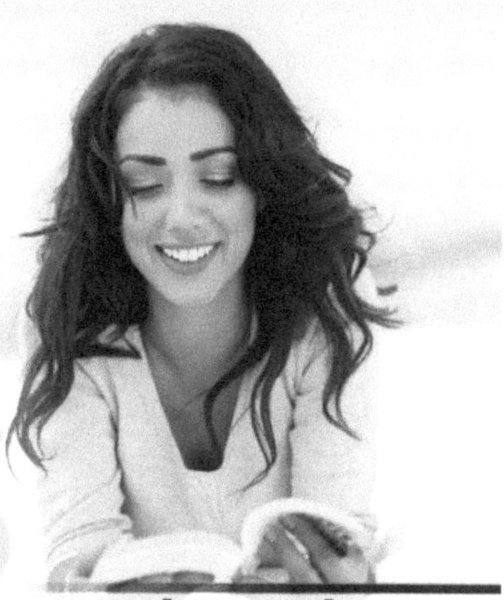

I want morebooks!

Buy your books fast and straightforward online - at one of world's fastest growing online book stores! Environmentally sound due to Print-on-Demand technologies.

Buy your books online at

www.morebooks.shop

Kaufen Sie Ihre Bücher schnell und unkompliziert online – auf einer der am schnellsten wachsenden Buchhandelsplattformen weltweit! Dank Print-On-Demand umwelt- und ressourcenschonend produzi ert.

Bücher schneller online kaufen

www.morebooks.shop

info@omniscriptum.com
www.omniscriptum.com

OMNIScriptum

FSC
www.fsc.org
MIX
Papier | Fördert gute Waldnutzung
FSC® C083411

Kolibri 360 GmbH
Ferdinand-Jühlke-Straße 7
99095 Erfurt, Deutschland
produktsicherheit@kolibri360.de

Druck:
CPI Druckdienstleistungen GmbH
im Auftrag der
Kolibri 360 GmbH
Ferdinand-Jühlke-Str. 7
99095 Erfurt